'With children's food marketing being so powerful, present, persuasive, and pernicious, it is essential that its effects be documented, mechanisms be understood, and means for prevention and mitigation be examined. This volume takes important steps in these directions by assembling state-of-the-art knowledge by leading experts in the field. It is a welcome advance.'

— **Prof. Dr. Kelly Brownell**, Director of the World Food Policy Center; Professor of Public Policy, Duke University, US.

'Seldom is social science as eye-opening as this volume. It is a riveting, evidence-based, collection on the avoidable public health epidemic of childhood obesity that, if unchecked, will result in significant personal and societal risks and costs. Through mainstream and online media, children are exposed to direct and subconscious inducements to consume snacks and drinks with extraordinary amounts of sugar, salt and fats. With evidence suggesting that industry self-regulation is ineffective, other solutions are discussed including legislation, nudging, promoting advertising literacy and a novel inhibition training approach. The volume is a timely call for action.'

— **Prof. Dr. George Gaskell**, Professor of Social Psychology, London School of Economics and Political Science, UK.

'Obesity has become an omnipresent health problem. This must-read book gives a critical and eclectic reflection on food marketing and its effect on children, adolescents, and adults. In *The Psychology of Food Marketing and (Over)eating* an unprecedented collection of research on food advertising and its effect on eating behavior is presented. This book clearly aims to promote healthy food marketing and gives students, researchers, health professionals, policy-makers, and dieticians a tool to change the world by promoting healthy eating behavior.'

— **Prof. Dr. Marjolijn Antheunis**, Tilburg University, School of Humanities and Digital Sciences, Netherlands.

'Food marketing is currently omnipresent, taking many forms and targeting people on a great variety of media platforms. This state of the art collection of chapters by key experts in the international field, from multiple perspectives, gives an eclectic overview on the effects of this extensive food marketing for unhealthy foods and what can be done about it in order to improve the health of children, adolescents, and adults.'

— **Prof. Dr. Moniek Buijzen**, Radboud University, Behavioural Science Institute, Netherlands.

THE PSYCHOLOGY OF FOOD MARKETING AND (OVER)EATING

Integrating recent research and existing knowledge on food marketing and its effects on the eating behaviour of children, adolescents and adults, this timely collection explores how food promotion techniques can be used to promote healthier foods.

Numerous factors influence what, when and how we eat, but one of the main drivers behind the unhealthy dietary intake of people is food marketing. Bringing together important trends from different areas of study, with state-of-the-art insights from multiple disciplines, the book examines the important factors and psychological processes that explain the effects of food marketing in a range of contexts, including social media platforms. The book also provides guidelines for future research by critically examining interventions and their effectiveness in reducing the impact of food marketing on dietary intake, in order to help develop new research programmes, legislation and techniques on what can be done about unhealthy food marketing.

With research conducted by leading scholars from across the world, this is essential reading for students and academics in psychology and related areas, as well as professionals interested in food marketing and healthy eating.

Dr. Frans Folkvord is an assistant professor at Tilburg School of Humanities and Digital Sciences, at the Department of Communication and Cognition, Tilburg University, The Netherlands. He is also a senior policy researcher at Open Evidence, a spin-off company of the Applied Social Science and Behavioral Economics Research group, University of Cataluña (Barcelona, Spain). He is a temporary advisor to the World Health Organization, UNICEF, European Commission, the Dutch Heart Foundation and the Dutch Nutrition Centre about the effects of food marketing on children's eating behaviour.

Current Issues in Social Psychology

Series Editor: Johan Karremans

Current Issues in Social Psychology is a series of edited books that reflect the state of current and emerging topics of interest in social psychology.

Each volume is tightly focused on a particular topic and consists of seven to ten chapters contributed by international experts. The editors of individual volumes are leading figures in their areas and provide an introductory overview.

The series is useful reading for students, academics and researchers of social psychology and related disciplines. Example topics include: self-esteem, mindfulness, evolutionary social psychology, minority groups, social neuroscience, cyberbullying and social stigma.

Mindfulness in Social Psychology
Edited by Johan C. Karremans and Esther K. Papies

Belief Systems and the Perception of Reality
Edited by Bastiaan Rutjens and Mark Brandt

Current Directions in Ostracism, Social Exclusion and Rejection Research
Edited by Selma Rudert, Rainer Greifeneder and Kipling Williams

New Directions in the Psychology of Close Relationships
Edited by Dominik Schoebi and Belinda Campos

The Psychology of Food Marketing and (Over)eating
Edited by Frans Folkvord

THE PSYCHOLOGY OF FOOD MARKETING AND (OVER)EATING

Edited by Frans Folkvord

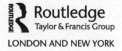

Routledge
Taylor & Francis Group

LONDON AND NEW YORK

First published 2020
by Routledge
2 Park Square, Milton Park, Abingdon, Oxon OX14 4RN

and by Routledge
52 Vanderbilt Avenue, New York, NY 10017

Routledge is an imprint of the Taylor & Francis Group, an informa business

British Library Cataloguing-in-Publication Data
A catalogue record for this book is available from the British Library

Library of Congress Cataloging-in-Publication Data
A catalog record has been requested for this book

ISBN: 978-0-367-22314-4 (hbk)
ISBN: 978-0-367-22316-8 (pbk)
ISBN: 978-0-429-27440-4 (ebk)

Typeset in Bembo
by Swales & Willis Ltd, Exeter, Devon, UK

Printed and bound by CPI Group (UK) Ltd, Croydon, CR0 4YY

CONTENTS

FOREWORD

Dr. Tim Lobstein

WORLD OBESITY FEDERATION, LONDON, UK

There is increasing recognition that the world's food supply system is malfunctioning. Recent estimates of the combined effects of undernutrition, excess bodyweight and poor dietary quality show that these consequences of a failing food supply are responsible for more ill health and premature death than any other single cause (1).

The failure of the food system is in part driven by the same forces that have led to its remarkable achievements over the past century, namely the cost efficiencies imposed on the supply chain by the drive for returns on investment. Mechanised production of long-shelf-life foods and beverages from basic commodities – starches, sugars, fats and oils – enhanced with flavourings and colourings increasingly dominates the low-cost end of the market. As the markets mature, these drives for efficiency are dominated by competitive marketing and brand promotion, led by product advertising. Advertising provides the essential link between the products of a competitive food supply chain and the creation of demand for the resulting products.

There are two direct purposes to advertising. One is to provide information to potential purchasers about a product. This is the purpose that is highly defended by the advertisers as being their right to exercise freedom of speech and to ensure the efficient operation of the marketplace. The other, arguably more significant, purpose is to induce positive feelings about a product so that potential purchasers view the product as desirable and attractive. This second role is more contentious as it works largely at an unconscious, subliminal level, and operates outside the classical market assumption of a purchaser making a purely rational choice.

Advertising depends on the creation of brands and logos to identify a unique, privately owned product. A company making chocolate has only a limited interest in promoting the sales of chocolate generally, including that of their competitors. They have a much greater interest in selling the chocolate that they themselves are manufacturing, and not their competitors', and therefore need to identify their own products by branding them. Other cues such as uniquely coloured packaging and labelling and associated cartoon characters, personalities and promotional gifts will also be used: but it is the brand that is key, and will be copyrighted, trade-marked and patented to defend its use.

Besides advertising messages to promote a product other techniques are used to encourage sales. The classic 'Four Ps' of product marketing include advertising (i.e. *promotion*), and also *pricing* (including discounts and special offers), *positioning* (both literally where it sits on a shelf or in a shop, as well as in comparison with other products in the same market space) and the *product* itself – its formulation and packaging and, in the case of food, ingredients such as colourings and flavourings to enhance desirability.

With the rapid increase in diet-related diseases in the late 20th century, and the highly visible rise in the numbers of people, including children, suffering excess bodyweight, there has been an increase in calls for a reduction in the consumption of unhealthy food products. It was summarised in the food trade journal *Food Navigator* in the simple headline *'"Eat less" – a difficult message for industry'* (2).

For consumers to eat less (and to eat more healthily), small changes are achievable through reformulation of popular products, along with the introduction of new products, and the reduction of product portion sizes. This works on the product element of the Four Ps. More radical policies include restricting the opportunities for discounted pricing and for advantageous positioning, and controlling the extent of promotional advertising.

Individual companies are understandably reluctant to restrict their own sales while other companies do not do so, and collective action by companies to control the market may be contrary to competition law. It follows that the most effective policies to limit promotional marketing will be industry-wide regulatory controls, whether operated by industry trade associations or by government agencies, and preferably backed by statutory powers of enforcement to prevent unfair competitive advantages.

When contemplating restrictions to promotional marketing, two approaches are available. The first is the principled, 'rights-based' approach, which at its core suggests that people, primarily children, should be protected from commercially driven inducements to consume (and over-consume). On the basis that children should not be considered rational consumers, it is argued that they should not be exposed to promotional marketing. In this approach, regulations are enacted to define the child and the child's rights.

The second approach is the 'risk-based' approach, which suggests that the market has freedoms that should only be curtailed on evidence of harm. With this approach, regulations need to define the victim of the harm, the degree of exposure to harm through the marketing, the nature of the marketing which induces harmful behaviour, the media used, and particularly the specific products which cause the harm.

While several countries have adopted rights-based approaches to the protection of children (notably in Scandinavia and in the province of Quebec, Canada), the risk-based approach is far more widespread but suffers from country-to-country variations in the definitions of vulnerability, exposure and harm, e.g. on the age of the child, the measures of exposure, the media used and the products to be restricted, and the type of regulatory authority responsible for enforcement.

Industry self-regulation, through industry-nominated and government-approved agencies, is favoured by many governments, and has been widely promoted in several regions. However, self-regulatory codes of practice such as the European Pledge (3) have been criticised for being slowly introduced, failing to cover all companies, poorly enforced with only weak sanctions available, and ultimately voluntary, and therefore easily reversed (4).

Both self-regulation and the more robust statutory regulations introduced by some countries have depended on definitions of the nature of the risk that exposes children to potential harm. Advances have been made in the research community to develop tools to aid policy making, principal amongst which is the development of nutrient-profiling tools that can define whether an individual food product is potentially harmful and so should be restricted in its marketing. Nutrient profiling began with moves in the 1990s to extend national recommendations for health from nutrient-based guidelines (vitamins, minerals, protein, etc.) to food-based guidelines (fruit and vegetables, meat and dairy, etc.). Food-based guidelines could then be used to define which foods contributed to improving health and which contributed to undermining health, based on their nutrient content, for example, on their content of dietary fibre, saturated fats, free sugars and sodium (salt).

Countries, and individual food and beverage companies, have adopted different profiling schemes for their own purposes. To some extent, variation between regions should be expected as national cuisines differ across the globe. To help normalise nutrient profiling the World Health Organization (WHO) is developing regional schemes which countries can use for their own regulation: as of early 2019 there are published schemes available for five of the six WHO regions (see Box). The use of nutrient-profiling schemes is a major technical advance, able to counter the common assertion by the food industry that 'there is no such thing as an unhealthy food, only an unhealthy diet'. Nutrient profiling is a powerful tool, able to define foods which should or should not be promoted for a range of purposes, e.g. for warnings on food labels, for school food services, for national food procurement policies and for government-funded research priorities (for more examples see McColl et al. (5)).

The availability of tools such as nutrient-profiling schemes has greatly assisted in the development of policies to control marketing to children, but the availability of such tools is not in itself enough. Like any regulation concerning commercial activity, policies to impose restrictions on marketing are likely to suffer from 'policy inertia' in getting proposed, designed, implemented and enforced. The policy inertia stems from several sources, including resistance from legislators due to their political ideology based on the maintenance of market freedoms, resistance from commercial interests protecting those freedoms, and a lack of public demand putting political pressure on legislators and consumer pressure on companies.

These sources of inertia can be countered by extending and refining the evidence base. High-quality evidence that relates directly to policy making can help support policy makers willing to contemplate change. Such evidence can also challenge companies over their voluntary measures when these are found inadequate. And evidence can stimulate public demand, for example by turning parents' anxiety over what their children eat into anger over what their children are being sold, and from there to public action to achieve change.

The Director-General of the UN's Food and Agriculture Organization, Dr José Graziano da Silva, has stated that the reason behind the increase in both hunger and obesity is that our food systems are not providing healthy diets. *'The current food systems do not work; they are designed for something other than guaranteeing good nutrition. Our challenge is to redesign them,'* he said (6). The purpose of advertising is to shape consumer demand to match the supply, and it follows that if the supply system is failing us, then action to control advertising is fully justified.

References

(1) Swinburn BA, Kraak VI, Allender S et al. The global syndemic of obesity, undernutrition and climate change: *The Lancet* commission report. *Lancet;* published online 27 January 2019. https://doi.org/10.1016/S0140-6736(18)32822-8 (accessed 25 March 2019).

(2) Scott-Thomas C. Eat less – a difficult message for industry. *foodnavigator-usa.com*, 7 February 2011. https://www.foodnavigator-usa.com/Article/2011/02/07/Eat-less-A-difficult-message-for-industry (accessed 25 March 2019).

(3) Anon. *EU pledge*. World Federation of Advertisers, 2019. www.eu-pledge.eu (accessed 25 March 2019).

(4) Harris JL, Pomeranz JL, Lobstein T, Brownell KD. A crisis in the marketplace: How food marketing contributes to childhood obesity and what can be done. *Annu Rev Public Health.* 2009;**30**:211–225.

(5) McColl K, Lobstein T, Brinsden H. Nutrient profiling could be used to transform food systems and support health-promoting food policies. World Health Organization: *Public Health Panorama*, 2017;4(3):586–597. http://www.euro.who.int/__data/assets/pdf_file/0018/357300/PHP-1124-NutrientProfiling-eng.pdf (accessed 25 March 2019).

(6) Graziano da Silva J. Deep shift in food systems needed to ensure healthy diets. Office of the Director-General, United Nations Food and Agriculture Organization: *Media release*, 15 January 2019. http://www.fao.org/news/story/en/item/1176876/icode/ (accessed 25 March 2019).

DEFINING FOODS AND BEVERAGES SUITABLE FOR MARKETING RESTRICTIONS

The World Health Organization (WHO) has provided technical support for the development of 'nutrient profile' models which allow food products to be categorised as suitable or not suitable for promotion to children. Five of the six WHO regions have published regional nutrient profile models:

- WHO Regional Office for Europe (2015) http://www.euro.who.int/__ data/assets/pdf_file/0005/270716/Nutrient-children_web-new.pdf
- Pan-American Health Organization/WHO Regional Office for the Americas (2016) http://iris.paho.org/xmlui/bitstream/handle/123456789/18621/ 9789275118733_eng.pdf
- WHO Regional Office for the Western Pacific (2016) http://apps.who.int/ iris/bitstream/handle/10665/252082/9789290617853-eng.pdf
- WHO Regional Office for South-East Asia (2017) http://apps.who.int/iris/ bitstream/handle/10665/253459/9789290225447-eng.pdf
- WHO Regional Office for the Eastern-Mediterranean (2017) http://apps. who.int/iris/bitstream/handle/10665/255260/EMROPUB_2017_en_19632. pdf

INTRODUCTION

Dr. Frans Folkvord

The current book will examine scientific research and public policy issues regarding food advertising and its effect on eating behavior. Food companies are among the largest promoters and marketers of their brands and products in the mainstream mass media and on other major promotional online platforms, aiming to increase their sales. While one of the most serious and persistent global health problems facing the world today is to make sure that people eat a healthy diet, food companies advertise for energy-dense and nutrition-poor foods, and only seldom for nutrition-rich foods.

It is widely acknowledged that obesity has emerged as an epidemic in the developed countries, starting around 1980 in the so-called "Western countries," spreading to other countries in the following decades. Currently, it is considered to be one of the biggest health concerns globally by national governments and international health institutes. An important factor that causes obesity is the over-consumption of energy-dense snacks that contains high levels of fat, sugar, and salt. Moreover, the increased intake of these unhealthy food products is considered as an important contributing factor of multiple chronic diseases, such as cardiovascular disease, diabetes, and multiple forms of cancer. In addition, this unhealthy dietary intake is repeatedly associated with negative mental well-being. So, in general, these energy-dense snacks make people sick and overweight. But why do people keep eating them then?

Numerous factors influence what, when, and how we eat, but one of the main drivers behind the unhealthy dietary intake of people over the world is food marketing. Food companies' marketing strategies target determinants for why people choose to eat one food rather than another, or more instead of less. In order to do that, food marketing is ubiquitous, to increase sales and comply with the laws of capitalism: increase profits to improve the value of the shares to satisfy the shareholders. It occurs in broadcast, digital, cinema, packaging, promotions, positioning in supermarkets, sponsorship, and in outdoor spaces. The industry spends billions to market their brands and products in an attempt to induce consumption behavior. Food cues of brands and products that are advertised are integrated in a great variety of (social) media platforms in an effort to create positive associations with these particular brands and products. As a consequence, whether unintended or not, people are (over)eating energy-dense foods worldwide.

In this book, we define marketing broadly: it includes activities and processes designed to communicate and deliver value to consumers, based on the general definition that has been stated by the American Marketing Association. This definition includes advertising (e.g., through purchased media, such as television, internet, radio), earned media (e.g., social media marketing, influencer marketing, public relations), promotions, and retail strategies. Therefore, food marketing is in this book considered as the communication to the consumer through a range of marketing techniques in order to add value to a food product and/or brand to persuade the consumer to purchase the product and/or brand.

The general aim of this book is to integrate recent research in food marketing with important recent and relevant insights regarding societal and political developments, and provide a guideline for future research, conducted by leading scholars from a great variety of disciplines (e.g., social and developmental psychology, marketing, nutrition and food science, human nutrition and health, law, and communication science). As a result, it will lead to an overview of state-of-the-art insights and guides the reader to important novel research areas that will be the future in this area. Currently, multiple societal developments, like the obesity-epidemic and the development of chronic diseases due to an unhealthy dietary intake, ask for an overview of the influence of food marketing on food consumption behavior. A book on this topic is thus highly needed and will bring together a set of important chapters.

Goal of this book

The specific goal of the book is to serve as an (a) overview of the existing knowledge with regard to food marketing and its effects on eating behavior of children, adolescents, and adults, and (b) a point of departure for the development of new research programs, legislation, and techniques about what can be done about unhealthy food marketing. This will be of use to graduate students and established researchers from a great variety of disciplines, health professionals, policy makers, dieticians, and nutritionists, and people who are interested in eating behavior.

We aim to achieve these goals by offering three book sections. *First*, we will provide chapters that summarize cutting-edge research by worldwide acknowledged experts in that specific area, thereby focusing on a selection of important factors and psychological processes that are found essential for explaining the effects of food marketing on children, adolescents, and adults. This approach acknowledges that food marketing is designed to target different age groups and explains the differences in techniques, effects, and individual susceptibility to food marketing. For example, in *Chapter 1* we will primarily address the extent, nature, and effects of broadcast and digital food marketing to young children, including an exploration of traditional and contemporary psychological theories that may explain some of the observed behavioral effects. The literature on broadcast food marketing is robust and shows that advertising of products which are high in fat, salt, and sugar increases children's consumption, preferences, and requests for these products. However there are fewer studies on digital food marketing. This research is important, as digital media is now children's primary and preferred form of media. Types of digital food marketing which will be covered are food brand websites, advergames, targeted advertisements, and social media marketing. On social media, marketers use direct and indirect avenues to promote their products. Direct forms of marketing include strategic placement of adverts both in and around social media, and food brand social media pages. Indirect forms include electronic word-of-mouth marketing via peers, social influencers, and celebrities. Thus digital food marketing is far more complex than broadcast and enables marketers to target children using subtler techniques, most of which children may not be aware of and therefore can be considered as unethical marketing practices.

Acknowledging young children's limited ability to recognize and defend against unwanted persuasive attempts, the food and beverage industry has established voluntary self-regulatory programs to limit unhealthy food marketing to children under 12 in countries worldwide. However, at the same time companies have increased marketing of unhealthy products, including sugary drinks, fast food, candy, and snacks to adolescents and young adults. Therefore, *Chapter 2* will focus on older youth, who tend to be highly skeptical of marketing, and they are also highly vulnerable to marketing influences, albeit in different ways. For example, their still-developing brains are highly responsive to reward cues and emotional messages; and their developmental need to establish separate identities leads them to value peer opinions and act to portray a socially desirable image. Many common food marketing techniques take advantage of these vulnerabilities, including social media marketing, celebrity endorsements, sports and music sponsorships, and influencer marketing. In addition, marketing disguised as entertainment content (e.g., video games, movies, TV shows, music) is designed to hide the persuasive intent of these messages and circumvent skeptical responses. In this chapter, common food marketing techniques used to target adolescents and young adults and the psychological processes that make young people highly vulnerable to their influence will be discussed.

Second, multiple chapters will focus on possible newly developed interventions and their effectiveness at reducing the impact of food marketing on dietary intake. These include legislation, inhibition training to reduce cue reactivity, and increasing advertising literacy. In *Chapter 3*, for example, we will discuss that food marketing to children has a negative impact on a broad range of their rights. States have a duty under the Convention on the Rights of the Child (CRC) to ensure that children's rights are effectively protected. One of the main advantages of a children's rights approach is to increase the accountability of States that do not respect their obligations under the CRC. To fulfill their obligations under the CRC, States should implement the World Health Organization (WHO) set of recommendations on the marketing of foods and non-alcoholic beverages to children. To implement the WHO recommendations effectively, States should adopt a comprehensive approach regulating both exposure to and power of marketing to limit its overall impact on children. In particular, they need to ensure that the focus moves from narrow definitions (of what constitutes a child or marketing to children) to limit the risk of investment shifts. Business actors have a responsibility (though not a legal obligation) to respect children's rights and should ensure that they do not promote unhealthy food to children, closing the loopholes in existing pledges / voluntary commitments.

In addition, *Chapter 4* describes that there are two major approaches towards protecting children from food marketing. The first takes a socio-environmental approach and seeks to reduce children's exposure to, and the power of, unhealthy food marketing by altering the media environment. The second is aimed at reducing the impact that marketing has on individuals, by focusing on behavioral or interpersonal solutions. To support regulatory controls, in 2010 the WHO released a set of recommendations to guide countries in restricting children's exposure to unhealthy food marketing and its power. These recommendations emphasize the important leadership role of governments in policy implementation and evaluation. Despite this, the predominant response to this issue globally has been in the implementation of self-regulatory codes of practice, developed and enforced by the food and advertising industries. Such codes may reflect good corporate responsibility, but, more likely, are a means of diverting industry criticism and impeding government regulations. This chapter will explore the range of regulatory responses globally to limit the exposure and power of food marketing, including showcasing best-practice examples, and the evidence on the effectiveness, or otherwise, of curbing marketing exposure, power, and impact.

Next, *Chapter 5* elaborates on children's sensitivity to food advertising, which has been the subject of social and political debate for many years. Besides concerns over the negative side effects of food advertising on the wellbeing of children, there are also concerns about the honesty of advertising targeted at children. The biggest concern is that children are not yet capable of critically assessing advertising. In comparison with adults, children are thought to be more vulnerable when confronted with advertising and, consequently, more sensitive to its impact. The rationale behind this common assumption is that the understanding of persuasion has not fully developed in children, and that therefore they are less capable of recognizing the temptations of advertising and evaluate it in a critical manner. In the children and advertising literature, these skills are often referred to as advertising literacy. In this chapter we will discuss how children's advertising literacy develops with age, the role of advertising literacy in children's susceptibility to food advertising, and how media education can increase children's advertising literacy skills and empower them to deal with food advertising.

Chapter 6 shows that food choices are mostly learned, and that preferences for food are for a large part shaped by pleasant or aversive experiences with food. After learning, mere perception of food items may elicit strong approach or avoidance reactions toward these foods relatively independently of intentions to eat these foods, which may cause difficulties with adhering to a healthy diet. This raises the question whether associations with food items can be changed to ultimately change food preferences. In this chapter, we will first discuss basic learning mechanisms that shape food preferences via the creation of pavlovian biases. In our culture these learning mechanisms tend to favor the development of preferences for higher-calorie foods rather than for lower-calorie foods. Then we will discuss recent work suggesting that such pavlovian biases favoring higher-calorie foods over lower-calorie foods may be reduced by associating food items with motor responses, or the absence thereof, during short computer trainings. We will outline how this approach may ultimately help consumers to choose foods they want.

Third, we will examine whether, when, and how food promotion techniques can be used to promote healthier foods, for example fruit and vegetables. In addition, we propose a new theoretical framework in *Chapter 7* that aims to explain the exact mechanism behind the promotion of healthier foods, that will set the research agenda for the upcoming decade(s) of scientific research in this area. Systematic reviews and experimental studies have repeatedly shown that food promotion for energy-dense foods stimulates unhealthy eating behavior among children. Moreover, most food promotion techniques target automatic process and focus on the rewarding aspects of palatable food products, inducing snack intake subconsciously. Due to the effectiveness of these food promotion activities children consume too much energy-dense foods and not enough healthy foods, according to international dietary standards. Considering the effectiveness and success of food promotion of unhealthy foods, it is highly promising to examine *whether, how, when*, and *for whom* food promotion for healthier foods might increase the intake among children. Different empirical studies have been conducted that tested the effect of healthy food promotion, but an overarching theoretical model that explains and predicts these effects is missing and needed. This review describes recent studies that have tested the effect of healthy food promotion on children's eating behavior and aims to present an integration of empirical findings in a new theoretical framework, the *Healthy Food Promotion Model* that increases the understanding of the effects of healthy food promotion on eating behavior and that might also be used for future research in this area.

Reference

World Health Organization. (2012). *A framework for implementing the set of recommendations on the marketing of foods and non-alcoholic beverages to children*. Geneva, Switzerland: WHO Press.

1

FOOD MARKETING TO YOUNG CHILDREN

Anna Coates and Dr. Emma Boyland

Introduction

'Obesogenic food environments' are considered to be a key driver of increasing childhood obesity globally (Ng et al., 2014; Powell, Schermbeck, & Chaloupka, 2013; Swinburn et al., 2011; Wang & Lim, 2012). The promotional strategies used in the ubiquitous marketing of food and beverages high in fat, salt and/or sugar (hereafter referred to as "HFSS foods") significantly contribute to these environments (WHO, 2010) and substantial evidence demonstrates the impact on younger children's (12 years and under) dietary health (Boyland et al., 2016; Sadeghirad, Duhaney, Motaghipisheh, Campbell, & Johnston, 2016; WHO, 2016).

Children are viewed to be an important demographic target group by food marketers and are preferentially targeted to a greater extent than any other group (Linn, 2013; Montgomery, 2015). This is likely because children affect product sales in three ways (Story & French, 2004): (1) children have independent spending power (pocket money which is often spent on snacks and confectionery); (2) children influence family expenditure (parents who are accompanied by children to the supermarket are more likely to acquiesce to children's demands, which are predominantly for branded HFSS products); and (3) children become adults, who are not only responsible for their own purchasing, but likely that of a complete family of their own. If brand loyalty is achieved during childhood, then a brand may benefit financially from that individual over the person's full lifespan.

Young children have captured notable research interest due to concerns over their particular vulnerability to the effects of marketing (Ali, Blades, Oates, & Blumberg, 2009; Kelly, Vandevijvere, et al., 2015; Story & French, 2004). It is suggested that, unlike adults, young children are less cognitively able to understand the persuasive intent of advertising (Story & French, 2004), i.e. the knowledge that advertising presents the best attributes of a product (and withholds negative attributes) in order to encourage sales (Kunkel, 2001). Therefore, any advertising which is targeted towards children could be considered, on this basis, to be exploitative. Regulations tend to be designed to protect younger and not older children, but public health researchers have repeatedly called for government-led protection of *all* individuals as no one is immune to persuasive food marketing (WHO, 2018).

The World Health Organization (WHO) states that the impact of HFSS food marketing is a function of both the level of *exposure* (i.e. the reach and frequency of promotions) and the *power* (i.e. via the creative content of the message, e.g. design, execution and persuasive techniques) of that marketing to produce behavioural change (e.g. greater preference for the marketed product, increased consumption of unhealthy foods) (WHO, 2010). An overview of the evidence on the exposure, power and impact of broadcast marketing (i.e. television) and digital marketing (i.e. internet and social media) of HFSS foods to young children will be discussed.

In addition, traditional and contemporary psychological theories that may explain some of the observed behavioural effects will be explored, including Information Processing Approach (McGuire, 1976), Food Marketing Defense Model (Harris, Brownell, & Bargh, 2009) and Reactivity to Embedded Food Cues in Advertising Model (Folkvord, Anschütz, Boyland, Kelly, & Buijzen, 2016).

Television advertising of HFSS food

Exposure

Despite recent increases in children's digital media consumption, television remains popular with children (Federal Trade Commission, 2012; Ofcom, 2016). In the UK, children (7–11 years) watch an average of 22 hours (12 hours commercial) of television per week (Boyland et al., 2018). A study that explored food advertising on UK television showed that children see an average rate of 3.5 food and beverage adverts per hour and that adverts for non-core food were shown most frequently (1.9 adverts per hour) (Whalen, Harrold, Child, Halford, & Boyland, 2017). This same study showed that the most heavily advertised foods were fast-food items (15.4%), followed by generic supermarket adverts (10.7%) and sugar-sweetened beverages (7.7%).

Children's likely exposure to food advertising on television varies somewhat between countries (Kelly et al., 2010), but in any country is highly likely to involve exposure to a considerable amount of advertising of HFSS foods (Boyland, Harrold, Kirkham, & Halford, 2011; Kent & Pauzé, 2018; Royo-Bordonada et al., 2016). The most recent global study on television food advertising prevalence included data from Western Europe, North and South America, Asia and Australia (Kelly et al., 2010). Food adverts accounted for 11–29% of all adverts analysed. The majority (53–87%) of these adverts promoted HFSS foods and were predominantly shown during peak child viewing periods.

In contrast, and inconsistent with national dietary recommendations, studies show a lack of, or complete absence of, adverts promoting fruit or vegetables (Powell et al., 2013; Whalen et al., 2017). This imbalance is reflected in the sizeable budgets of the food industry in comparison to health campaigns. For example, a total of £143 million was spent by the largest HFSS product companies in the UK in 2017 (Obesity Health Alliance, 2017). This figure is 27 times larger than the amount that the UK Government spent on promoting healthy eating practices in the same year, estimated to be £5 million (Obesity Health Alliance, 2017).

Power

Promotional techniques used in HFSS food advertising are based on extensive market research by the food and advertising industries and differ depending on the target market (Schor & Ford, 2007). For instance, toy giveaways and movie tie-ins are often used in fast-food television marketing aimed at young audiences (Bernhardt, Wilking, Gottlieb, Emond, & Sargent, 2014) but are less apparent in equivalent marketing targeted at adults (Bernhardt, Wilking, Adachi-Mejia, Bergamini, & Marijnissen, 2013). Frequently used techniques when marketing to children are premium offers (e.g. free gift, competitions and vouchers), promotional characters, celebrity endorsers, nutritional and health claims, and themes of 'taste' and of 'fun' (Boyland, Harrold, Kirkham, & Halford, 2012; Jenkin, Madhvani, Signal, & Bowers, 2014).

Due to regulatory pressures, HFSS food manufacturers are increasingly engaging in a variety of health-promoting marketing initiatives (Sütterlin & Siegrist, 2015), such as positioning HFSS products in the context of a 'healthy and balanced diet' (Harris, Haraghey, Lodolce, & Semenza, 2018). One study identified foods featured in television advertisements as either 'primary' (the focus of the advert) or 'incidental' and found that, when featured, incidental foods tended to be healthier than primary foods (Adams, Tyrrell, & White, 2011).

Another initiative is the use of health-related messaging. Implicit health claims (depiction of physical activity) and explicit health claims (health and nutritional messages), which one would expect to be used in promotion of healthy foods, were found most commonly in adverts promoting HFSS foods (Whalen, Harrold, Child, Halford, & Boyland, 2018). Marketers assert that depicting HFSS products in this way encourages children to maintain healthy lifestyles. However, research suggests they lead children to misinterpret foods (Bernhardt et al., 2014) and make poor judgements when making healthy food choices (Harris et al., 2018). For example, children who were shown a television advert for an HFSS breakfast cereal which depicted physical activity perceived the cereal as being healthier than children who were shown the same advert with no physical activity depicted (Castonguay, 2015). Also, children (7–10 years) exposed to adverts promoting 'healthy' fast-food meal options (e.g. McDonald's Happy Meal with a fruit pack and mineral water) showed increased liking of fast food in general but did not choose healthier meal options from a fast-food menu (Boyland, Kavanagh-Safran, & Halford, 2015).

Impact

The impact of television HFSS food advertising on determinants of eating and children's actual eating behaviour has been assessed using a multitude of behavioural measures. The range of outcomes of interest were conceptualised by Kelly et al. (2015) in the model shown in Figure 1.1; examples from many of these steps will be drawn for consideration in the current chapter.

Food, as a commodity, is one of the most highly branded items (Story & French, 2004). Food marketing often takes a brand-centred approach in order to build brand awareness and loyalty (Heath, 2009). From a very young age children display HFSS food brand awareness. An Australian study found that 76% of children (5–12 years) correctly matched at least one sport to the correct HFSS brand sports sponsor (Pettigrew, Rosenberg, Ferguson, Houghton, & Wood, 2013), which is concerning given that many sports events and teams are sponsored by fast-food companies. Brand awareness is an antecedent of brand preference, and children are shown to prefer the taste of foods served in branded packaging (McDonald's wrapping) in comparison with identical foods served in unbranded packaging (Robinson, Borzekowski, Matheson, & Kraemer, 2007). Children also prefer HFSS food brands that are endorsed by celebrities (Boyland et al., 2013; Smits, Vandebosch, Neyens, & Boyland, 2015) and have more positive attitudes towards foods featured in television adverts than those that are not (Boyland et al., 2016; Dixon, Scully, Wakefield, White, & Crawford, 2007; Sadeghirad et al., 2016).

A review of studies looking at the effect of HFSS food advertising on children's product requests found that the majority showed exposure increased requests for advertised products (McDermott, O'Sullivan, Stead, & Hastings, 2006). Importantly, a large-scale study using data from eight European countries linked children's (2–9 years) requests for HFSS foods to overall diet and body weight (Huang et al., 2016). Specifically, children who 'often' requested these items were 31% more likely to have overweight (when weighed at a 2-year follow-up) than children who 'never' requested products, suggesting that overweight children may be more susceptible to food advertising than normal-weight children (Russell, Croker, & Viner, 2018). Collectively these studies demonstrate how HFSS food advertising contributes to children's poorer dietary health. Parents would support changes to the 'obesogenic food environment' that could lessen instances of 'pester power', including reducing children's exposure to HFSS food advertising and positioning these products out of children's eyeline in supermarkets (Henry & Borzekowski, 2011).

Advertising also influences how children spend their own money. Children (aged 7–11) in the UK who watched a minimum of 3 hours of television per day were almost three times more likely to buy HFSS foods with pocket money and were over twice as likely to report consumption of HFSS foods compared

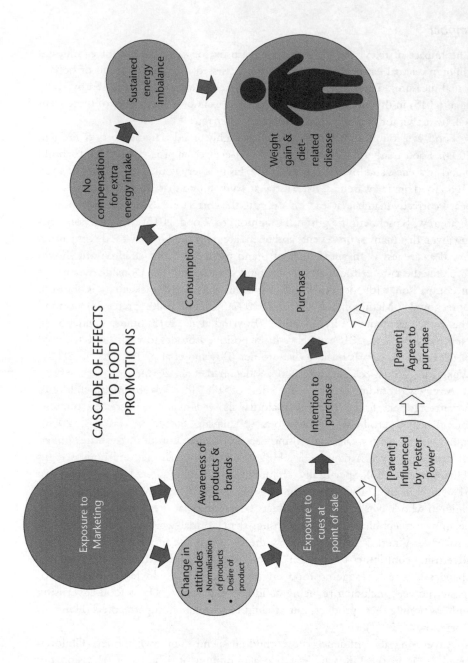

FIGURE 1.1 A schematic model of the multi-level impacts of children's exposure to unhealthy food marketing (Kelly et al., 2015).

with children who watched minimal or no television (Boyland et al., 2018). Food intake is arguably the most appropriate and relevant outcome measure related to weight gain. Several meta-analyses have experimentally manipulated food advertising exposure (exposure vs. no exposure), both on television and the internet, and measured immediate post-exposure intake. They concluded that exposure significantly increased overall food intake (Boyland et al., 2016; Sadeghirad et al., 2016) and that younger children (under 8 years) had increased calorie intake compared with older children (Sadeghirad et al., 2016). In terms of effect on overall diet, children (10–16 years) in the US who watched commercial television were found to have nutritionally poorer diets than those who watched non-commercial television (Kelly et al., 2016). Recently it has been demonstrated that increased food intake as a response to food marketing exposure was not compensated for at a subsequent meal, supporting the notion that this increased consumption would, over time, lead to weight gain (Norman et al., 2018).

Digital marketing of HFSS food

Exposure

Digital marketing is defined as 'promotional activity, delivered through a digital medium, that seeks to maximise impact through creative and/or analytical methods' (WHO, 2016). Digital platforms collect personal information on users to deliver advertising which is targeted, engaging and encourages users to share experiences with peers (WHO, 2016). Marketing in this medium is less overt than on traditional media, meaning it likely bypasses any media literacy children may possess and amplifies the effects seen in television food advertising (Harris et al., 2009). Awareness of where children spend time online is critical to understanding both the nature and the quantity of digital food marketing they may be exposed to. Children in Westernised societies avidly access digital media, predominantly on personal mobile devices, and the most popular sites visited are those with mixed audience appeal such as social media (e.g. Facebook, Instagram, YouTube) (Statistica.com, 2018; WHO, 2016). The internet has advanced from being a space predominantly comprised of static websites to a more social and participatory space, providing marketers with further opportunities to target and interact with potential customers (Gensler, Völckner, Liu-Thompkins, & Wiertz, 2013). Capitalising on this evolution, food companies are increasingly using social media to market to children (Freeman et al., 2014).

In digital media, detailed analytics allow brands, marketers and platforms to identify the 'reach' of adverts as well as the attention received by them (Facebook for Business, 2015). Marketers are able to target children much more specifically than in traditional media as they are informed by analytics of users' emotions, behaviour, locations and even food consumption patterns (Holmberg, Chaplin, Hillman, & Berg, 2016; Kelly, Bochynska, Kornman, & Chapman, 2008). Food marketers assert that the use of analytics is positive for consumers in general, as consumers are only targeted with advertising which is considered 'relevant' to them (Turow, 2011). Others view these practices to be wholly unethical and take the view that the use of personal information to target marketing at individuals who may be particularly susceptible is 'unfair and deceptive' (Reidenberg, Breaux, Cranor, & French, 2015).

Social media (e.g. Facebook, Instagram, YouTube) is popular with young children (Ofcom, 2016), despite platforms generally requiring subscribed users to be a minimum age of 13 years. Many children access these platforms by subscribing with fake date of birth or using accounts set up by their parents (Ofcom, 2016). Research shows that, just like television advertising, the foods promoted on digital media are predominantly HFSS. A recent study analysed the frequency of in-video advertisements of food and beverages in the most popular YouTube videos targeted at children (Tan, See Hoe, Azahadi, & Tilakavati, 2018). In total 187 adverts were assessed, and the most common category was food and beverage adverts (38%). Just over half of these adverts promoted non-core (HFSS) foods, and the remainder promoted core (healthy) or miscellaneous items.

Consistent with these results, a study in Canada identified the top ten most popular websites with children (2–11 years) and determined the frequency of banner and pop-up adverts for food and beverages over a year (Kent & Pauzé, 2018). The nutritional quality of food adverts was assessed using the Pan American Health Organization and UK Nutrient Profile Models. Approximately 54 million adverts were viewed in total: the majority (93.4%) were promoted HFSS foods, or (73.8%) 'less healthy' foods according to the UK Nutrient Profile Model. These studies provide important illustrations of children's *potential* exposure to food marketing, but there are notable limitations in what these studies can tell us about their true exposure, for reasons that are discussed in brief below (for a more extensive discussion, see WHO 2016).

There are substantial methodological, ethical and legal challenges when measuring children's *actual* exposure to digital marketing of HFSS foods. Information on engagement with content is often restricted to providers and is costly to access (Kelly et al., 2015; Stevenson, 2014). In addition, behavioural target marketing means that content varies from person to person (Tatlow-Golden, Tracey, & Dolphin, 2016; WHO, 2016). Despite this, public health researchers have identified some useful means of illustrating the extent of children's exposure, such as the use of so-called 'avatar' studies. In these studies, hypothetical children's profiles were created on social media, portraying the children to have previously 'liked' HFSS food brands (Jenkin, Signal, & Smith, 2014; Vassallo et al., 2018). Over a few weeks, children received a high frequency of targeted and curated HFSS brand marketing via shared posts and paid advertisements.

Power

HFSS food marketing in digital media uses immersive techniques such as HFSS-themed advergames, user-created social media content, electronic word-of-mouth recommendations shared on social media via 'likes' and 'shares' and paid partnerships with celebrities and social media influencers (e.g. YouTube video bloggers).

Advergames are online games that feature branded messages, logos and/or characters and are developed by brands as a promotional tool (Mallinckrodt & Mizerski, 2007). Children are more likely to visit food brand websites with advergames than those without (Harris, Speers, Schwartz, & Brownell, 2012), and have unlimited access to them when online. Marketing of this nature is based on the premise that children associate the promoted brand with a positive experience as they play (Hernandez & Chapa, 2010). It is also typically less overt whereby food cues are highly embedded into engaging and entertaining content and children are actively encouraged to share these experiences with peers (Cheyne, Dorfman, Bukofzer, & Harris, 2013; Lawlor, Dunne, & Rowley, 2016).

On social media, marketers have children doing their job for them by prompting children to interact with adverts and propagate them through their peer networks. Children are encouraged to engage with marketing by 'hashtagging', 'liking' and 'sharing' posts made by brands and also 'subscribing' to content posted by brands (Gaber & Wright, 2014). For example, on Facebook users can become fans of food brands by 'liking' the brands page, which typically feature photos and videos uploaded by the brand and the fans (Harris et al., 2014). This activity is logged in the user's 'newsfeed' and in the newsfeeds of their peers. Polls are also used to introduce new products, gain product feedback and obtain information about customer preferences (Richardson & Harris, 2011). Users are even able to order takeaways without leaving the brand's social media page. Engagement beyond the brand's Facebook page is encouraged by suggesting that fans register via SMS or email to receive 'exclusive deals', coupons and offers. Research shows that HFSS food marketing that has the greatest reach with children used tactics of peer engagement, emotion and entertainment (Childwise, 2016).

Word-of-mouth recommendations shared on social media are considered to be a powerful form of marketing (Buchanan, Kelly, & Yeatman, 2017). Young people are shown to trust brand or product recommendations from peers more than those direct from a brand (Chu & Kim, 2011; Kim & Johnson, 2016). Food brands build engagement in social networks via 'seeding' messages on social media (Brown, Broderick, & Lee, 2007). These messages are then disseminated easily and rapidly amongst peers. For example, Coca-Cola launched a campaign in 2015 to make a personal connection with consumers (Mendoza, 2015). People's names were printed on bottle labels and the hashtag '*ShareaCoke*' was used to encourage social media users to share images of themselves drinking a Coke. Over one million more people consumed a Coca-Cola because of this campaign. Using social media in this way enables companies to have wider dissemination of their advertising messages (Kelly et al., 2015) with relatively less monetary investment compared to television advertising (WHO, 2013).

Food marketing via paid-for recommendations from celebrities and social media influencers is increasingly common (Kelly et al., 2015). Popstar Selena Gomez has over 100 million Instagram followers. In a recent campaign Coca-Cola paid her

$500,000 to post an image of herself sipping a bottle of Coca-Cola. This image received over six million 'likes' on Instagram (Heine, 2016).

In a recent survey by Google, 70% of young people reported they would be more influenced by a brand recommendation from their favourite YouTube video blogger than a movie or television personality (The Drum, 2018). Social media influencers (e.g. YouTube video bloggers) are popular with children (Ofcom, 2016) not only because their content is entertaining but also because of the information shared (Hsu & Tsou, 2011). Viewers tend to place more trust in the recommendations of those they feel close to and similar to, evident in the success of campaigns which use peer word-of-mouth recommendations (Berryman & Kavka, 2017; De Veirman, Cauberghe, & Hudders, 2017). The communication channels (e.g. 'like' and 'shares') enabled in social media help to create a sense of a bi-directional relationship between viewer and influencer, leading viewers to feel they know the influencer on a personal level, labelled as para-social interaction (Aladwani, 2014). Para-social interaction is the illusion of a relationship with a media character and is argued to make consumers more likely to follow their opinions (Knoll & Matthes, 2017). Despite the popularity of influencer marketing, scientifically grounded insights into why influencers are persuasive among children and which psychological mechanisms underlie their persuasive effect have not been explored in the context of digital food marketing.

Impact

Compared to television advertising, evidence of the impact of digital food marketing on behaviour is in its infancy – but it is increasing. Recent meta-analyses show that both television and digital food marketing affect young people's eating behaviour (Boyland et al., 2016; Folkvord & van 't Riet, 2018; Russell et al., 2018; Sadeghirad et al., 2016) These findings are not surprising given that food marketers themselves report that not only is digital marketing successful, it amplifies the effects of marketing in traditional media (Facebook for Business, 2015). A quantitative online survey of over 2400 parents and children (aged 7–11) in the UK found that children who used the internet for more than 3 hours per day were almost three times more likely to request that their parents buy HFSS foods, four times more likely to buy HFSS foods themselves, and consumed less fruit and vegetables, than children who used the internet for little or no time (Boyland et al., 2018).

Experimental data of the impact of advergames on children's food intake has received most attention when looking at the effect of digital food marketing. A set of studies by Folkvord and colleagues (Folkvord et al., 2017; Folkvord, Anschütz, Buijzen, & Valkenburg, 2013; Folkvord, Anschütz, Wiers, & Buijzen, 2015; Folkvord, Anschutz, Nederkoorn, Westerik, & Buijzen, 2014) demonstrated that advergames promoting HFSS food brands increased children's immediate overall intake compared with non-food advergames. In addition, research shows that even children as young as 8 years can display awareness of the persuasive intent of an advergame (Mallinckrodt & Mizerski, 2007). However, this awareness did not affect children's response to marketing, with children still found to prefer the promoted HFSS cereal brand Kellogg's Froot Loops to other brands of cereal.

An early theory of advertising, the Information Processing Approach (McGuire, 1976), asserted that knowledge of the persuasive intent of advertising helps children to counteract its effects. In addition, media literacy programmes have been developed as strategies to increase persuasion knowledge in children (e.g. industry-funded MediaSmart in the UK (http://www.mediasmart.org.uk). However, if persuasion knowledge is not associated with increased resistance to advertising, it is not clear what benefit these programmes could have in relation to helping children resist advertising's influence (Folkvord et al., 2017). In support, the Food Marketing Defense Model (Harris et al., 2009) states that four conditions must be met in order for children to counter the effects of food marketing: *awareness* of advertising, *understanding* of its persuasive intent, and the *ability* and *motivation* to resist. However, it could be argued that children are unlikely ever to be motivated to resist food marketing. Unlike adults, they are less driven by long-term goals such as health (Harris et al., 2018) and instead are more impulsive and driven by taste and hedonic preference for HFSS foods (Bruce et al., 2016).

The effect of social media food marketing has received very little research attention, but data are now beginning to emerge. A recent online survey in Australia examined whether online behaviours including social media use were associated with food and beverage consumption in children (10–16 years) (Baldwin, Freeman, & Kelly, 2018). Results demonstrated that seeing favourite food brands advertised online (e.g. Facebook sidebar advert), watching food brand video content (e.g. YouTube video posted by the brand) and making online food purchases (e.g. ordering takeaway food online) were all associated with a higher reported consumption of unhealthy food and drinks. These effects remained significant when adjusting for age, sex and socio-economic status and were increased in children with higher online engagement with food brands.

Another study tested the impact of social media influncer food marketing on children's (9–11 years) eating behaviour (Coates, Hardman, Halford, Christiansen, & Boyland, 2019). Children were divided into three groups and viewed Instagram profiles of popular influencers. Profiles featured images of the influencer holding unhealthy snacks, healthy snacks or non-food products. Afterwards, to measure food intake, children were offered plates of healthy and unhealthy snacks. Children who viewed images of influencers with unhealthy snack images consumed 32% more kilocalories (kcals) from unhealthy snacks specifically and 26% more kcals in total (from healthy and unhealthy snacks) compared with children who saw images of influencers with non-food products. There was no significant effect of viewing influencers with healthy snacks on children's kcal intake (healthy, unhealthy or total). These findings suggest that the marketing of unhealthy foods, via social media influencers, increases children's immediate energy intake.

These findings are supported by the Reactivity to Embedded Food Cues in Advertising Model (Folkvord et al., 2016), which suggests that the impact of food marketing is moderated by message factors, including the level of integration of food cues. While television advertising appears at recognisable intervals within and between programming often signalled by the presence of cues such as jingles or defined advert breaks (Owen, Lewis, Auty, & Buijzen, 2013), digital marketing is often embedded in the online content itself (Wright, Friestad, & Boush, 2005). Therefore food cues that are integrated into digital media content are processed with minimal cognitive elaboration (Buijzen, Van Reijmersdal, & Owen, 2010; Cauberghe & De Pelsmacker, 2010), diminishing children's ability to recognise when they are being advertised to (Freeman, Chapman, & Freeman, 2007; Rozendaal, Lapierre, van Reijmersdal, & Buijzen, 2011), and making this type of marketing more difficult to defend against.

Sustained impact of television and digital HFSS food marketing

Cohort studies indicate that an energy gap of 69–77 kcal per day is all that is required for a child to become overweight (Van Den Berg et al., 2011). Meta-analyses and systematic reviews of the impact of acute exposure to food advertising on television and in digital media indicate that in general it increases children's kcal intake by approximately 30–50 kcal (Boyland et al., 2016; Sadeghirad et al., 2016). These results are concerning because the majority of studies measure children's response to an acute exposure to advertising only. The effect may be much larger in real life (Gortmaker et al., 2011) due to the sheer extent of, and repeated exposure to, food marketing that children in Westernised societies are potentially exposed to on many platforms and in many different settings.

Unfortunately, children do not compensate for the increased intake of food due to exposure to food advertising by consuming less food at later meal occasions. A study conducted at children's (aged 7–12) summer camps in Australia looked at energy intake across the course of a day (Norman et al., 2018). Children were exposed to food marketing on television, on digital media, or both. Food consumption was measured immediately after exposure by snack intake, and also at lunch later in the day. Children exposed to food marketing consumed more at subsequent snack intake, and also did not reduce their intake at lunch later in the day (consuming an additional 194 kilojoules of energy overall), compared with children who saw non-food marketing. The effect was increased in children who saw marketing on both television and in digital media as opposed to just one medium. Therefore, HFSS food marketing contributes to a positive energy-gap which, over time, could lead to heavier weight.

Conclusion

Data from the US, Australia and Europe show that the quantity of advertising that a child is exposed to increases the likelihood of a child having overweight (Lobstein & Dibb, 2005). Children who are high commercial television viewers are associated with increased odds of 59% of having overweight or obesity compared with low commercial television viewers, and high internet use was associated with increased odds of 79% relative to low use (Boyland et al., 2018). Modelling studies have estimated that, if television advertisements of fast food were banned, obesity prevalence would be reduced by 14–18% (Chou & Grossman, 2008). In addition, digital marketing offers food companies new ways to reach children, which are difficult to monitor and the effects challenging to quantify (WHO, 2016). The borderless nature of the internet means that coordinated action is required globally to limit children's exposure to the marketing of unhealthy foods. This action is critical in order to inform better food choices, improve children's diets and prevent the increasing rates of childhood obesity seen globally.

Despite this evidence the food industry is critical of the lack of evidence that shows a direct link between children's exposure to HFSS food marketing and children's body weight. To establish a direct causal relationship between food marketing and (childhood) obesity, a randomised controlled experiment is needed for multiple years with a large group of children. However it is impossible to isolate a child from all factors, other than food marketing, to determine whether there is a causal effect. Weight gain is typically gradual (Kelly et al., 2015) and there are numerous environmental factors that children are exposed to which are known to influence weight (Lake & Townsend, 2006). It is likely that the pathway between HFSS food marketing exposure and children's body weight and associated health outcomes is complex (Kelly et al., 2015), but there is substantial and highly convincing evidence presented in this chapter on marketing's effect on a number of determinants of behavioural measures.

References

Adams, J., Tyrrell, R., & White, M. (2011). Do television food advertisements portray advertised foods in a "healthy" food context? *British Journal of Nutrition, 105*(6), 810–815. https://doi.org/10.1017/S0007114510004435

Aladwani, A. M. (2014). The 6As model of social content management. *International Journal of Information Management, 34*, 133–138. https://doi.org/10.1016/j.ijinfomgt.2013.12.004

Ali, M., Blades, M., Oates, C., & Blumberg, F. (2009). Young children's ability to recognize advertisements in web page designs. *The British Journal of Developmental Psychology, 27*(Pt 1), 71–83. https://doi.org/10.1348/026151008X388378

Baldwin, H. J., Freeman, B., & Kelly, B. (2018). Like and share: Associations between social media engagement and dietary choices in children. *Public Health Nutrition.* https://doi.org/10.1017/S1368980018001866

Bernhardt, A. M., Wilking, C., Adachi-Mejia, A. M., Bergamini, E., & Marijnissen, J. (2013). How television fast food marketing aimed at children compares with adult advertisements. *PLoS ONE, 8*(8), 72479. https://doi.org/10.1371/journal.pone.0072479

Bernhardt, A. M., Wilking, C., Gottlieb, M., Emond, J., & Sargent, J. D. (2014). Children's reaction to depictions of healthy foods in fast-food television advertisements. *JAMA Pediatrics, 168*(5), 422–426. https://doi.org/10.1001/jamapediatrics.2014.140

Berryman, R., & Kavka, M. (2017). 'I guess a lot of people see me as a big sister or a friend': The role of intimacy in the celebrification of beauty vloggers. *Journal of Gender Studies, 26*(3), 307–320. https://doi.org/10.1080/09589236.2017.1288611

Boyland, E. J., Harrold, J. A., Dovey, T. M., Allison, M., Dobson, S., Jacobs, M. C., & Halford, J. C. G. (2013). Food choice and overconsumption: Effect of a premium sports celebrity endorser. *Journal of Pediatrics*, *163*(2), 339–343. https://doi.org/10.1016/j.jpeds.2013.01.059

Boyland, E. J., Harrold, J. A., Kirkham, T. C., & Halford, J. C. G. (2011). The extent of food advertising to children on UK television in 2008. *International Journal of Pediatric Obesity*, *6*(5–6), 455–461. https://doi.org/10.3109/17477166.2011.608801

Boyland, E. J., Harrold, J. A., Kirkham, T. C., & Halford, J. C. G. (2012). Persuasive techniques used in television advertisements to market foods to UK children. *Appetite*, *58*(2), 658–664. https://doi.org/10.1016/j.appet.2011.11.017

Boyland, E. J., Kavanagh-Safran, M., & Halford, J. C. G. (2015). Exposure to "healthy" fast food meal bundles in television advertisements promotes liking for fast food but not healthier choices in children. *British Journal of Nutrition*, *113*(6), 1012–1018. https://doi.org/10.1017/S0007114515000082

Boyland, E. J., Nolan, S., Kelly, B., Tudur-Smith, C., Jones, A., Halford, J. C. G., & Robinson, E. (2016). Advertising as a cue to consume: A systematic review and meta-analysis of the effects of acute exposure to unhealthy food and nonalcoholic beverage advertising on intake in children and adults. *American Journal of Clinical Nutrition*, *103*(2), 519–533. https://doi.org/10.3945/ajcn.115.120022

Boyland, E., Whalen, R., Christiansen, P., Mcgale, L., Duckworth, J., Halford, J., . . . Vohra, J. (2018). *See it, want it, buy it, eat it: How food advertising is associated with unhealthy eating behaviours in 7–11 year old children.* Retrieved from http://www.cancerresearchuk.org/

Brown, J., Broderick, A. J., & Lee, N. (2007). Word of mouth communication within online communities: Conceptualizing the online social network. *Journal of Interactive Marketing.* https://doi.org/10.1002/dir.20082

Bruce, A. S., Pruitt, S. W., Ha, O.-R., Cherry, J. B. C., Smith, T. R., Bruce, J. M., & Lim, S.-L. (2016). The influence of televised food commercials on children's food choices: Evidence from ventromedial prefrontal cortex activations. *The Journal of Pediatrics*, *177*, 1–7. https://doi.org/10.1016/j.jpeds.2016.06.067

Buchanan, L., Kelly, B., & Yeatman, H. (2017). Exposure to digital marketing enhances young adults' interest in energy drinks: An exploratory investigation. *PLoS ONE*, *12*(2), 1–17. https://doi.org/10.1371/journal.pone.0171226

Buijzen, M., Van Reijmersdal, E. A., & Owen, L. H. (2010). Introducing the PCMC model: An investigative framework for young people's processing of commercialized media content. *Communication Theory*, *20*(4), 427–450. https://doi.org/10.1111/j.1468-2885.2010.01370.x

Castonguay, J. (2015). Portraying physical activity in food advertising targeting children. *Health Education*, *115*(6), 534–553. https://doi.org/10.1108/HE-07-2014-0080

Cauberghe, V., & De Pelsmacker, P. (2010). Advergames. The impact of brand prominence and game repetition on brand responses. *Journal of Advertising*, *39*(1), 5–18. https://doi.org/10.2753/JOA0091-3367390101

Cheyne, A. D., Dorfman, L., Bukofzer, E., & Harris, J. L. (2013). Marketing sugary cereals to children in the digital age: A content analysis of 17 child-targeted websites. *Journal of Health Communication*, *18*(5), 563–582. https://doi.org/10.1080/10810730.2012.743622

Childwise. (2016). *New CHILDWISE report reveals children's favourite internet vloggers.* Retrieved August 2, 2017, from http://www.childwise.co.uk/uploads/3/1/6/5/31656353/childwise_press_release_-_vloggers_2016.pdf

Chou, S.-Y., & Grossman, M. (2008). Fast-food restaurant advertising on television and its influence on childhood obesity. *Journal of Law and Economics* (Vol. 51). Retrieved from http://www.journals.uchicago.edu/t-and-c

Chu, S.-C., & Kim, Y. (2011). Determinants of consumer engagement in electronic word-of-mouth (eWOM) in social networking sites. *International Journal of Advertising, 31*(1), 47–75.

Coates, A. E., Hardman, C. A., Halford, J. C. G., Christiansen, P., & Boyland, E. J. (2019). Social media influencer marketing and children's food intake: A randomized trial. *Pediatrics, 143*(4), 1–9. https://doi.org/10.1542/peds.2018-2554

De Veirman, M., Cauberghe, V., & Hudders, L. (2017). Marketing through Instagram influencers: The impact of number of followers and product divergence on brand attitude. *International Journal of Advertising, 36*(5), 798–828. https://doi.org/10.1080/02650 487.2017.1348035

Dixon, H. G., Scully, M. L., Wakefield, M. A., White, V. M., & Crawford, D. A. (2007). The effects of television advertisements for junk food versus nutritious food on children's food attitudes and preferences. *Social Science & Medicine, 65*, 1311–1323. https://doi.org/10.1016/j.socscimed.2007.05.011

Facebook for Business. (2015). Introducing new ways to buy, optimise and measure ads for a mobile world. Retrieved July 30, 2018, from https://www.facebook.com/business/news/Ad-Week-UK

Federal Trade Commission. (2012). *A review of food marketing to children and adolescents follow-up report.* Retrieved from https://www.ftc.gov/sites/default/files/documents/reports/review-food-marketing-children-and-adolescents-follow-report/121221foodmarketing report.pdf

Folkvord, F., Anschütz, D. J., Boyland, E., Kelly, B., & Buijzen, M. (2016). Food advertising and eating behavior in children. *Current Opinion in Behavioral Sciences, 9*, 26–31. https://doi.org/10.1016/j.cobeha.2015.11.016

Folkvord, F., Anschütz, D. J., Buijzen, M., & Valkenburg, P. M. (2013). The effect of playing advergames promoting healthy or unhealthy foods on actual food intake among children. *The American Journal of Clinical Nutrition, 97*, 239–245. https://doi.org/10.1016/j.appet.2012.05.062

Folkvord, F., Anschutz, D., Nederkoorn, C., Westerik, H., & Buijzen, M. (2014). Impulsivity, "advergames," and food intake. *Pediatrics, 133*(6), 1007–1012. https://doi.org/10.1542/peds.2013-3384

Folkvord, F., Anschütz, D. J., Wiers, R. W., & Buijzen, M. (2015). The role of attentional bias in the effect of food advertising on actual food intake among children. *Appetite, 84*, 251–258. https://doi.org/10.1016/j.appet.2014.10.016

Folkvord, F., Lupiáñez-Villanueva, F., Codagnone, C., Bogliacino, F., Veltri, G., & Gaskell, G. (2017). Does a 'protective' message reduce the impact of an advergame promoting unhealthy foods to children? An experimental study in Spain and The Netherlands. *Appetite, 112*, 117–123. https://doi.org/10.1016/j.appet.2017.01.026

Folkvord, F., & van 't Riet, J. (2018). The persuasive effect of advergames promoting unhealthy foods among children: A meta-analysis. *Appetite.* https://doi.org/10.1016/j.appet.2018.07.020

Freeman, B., Chapman, S., & Freeman, M. B. (2007). Is '"YouTube"' telling or selling you something? Tobacco content on the YouTube video-sharing website. *Tobacco Control, 16*, 207–210. https://doi.org/10.1136/tc.2007.020024

Freeman, B., Kelly, B., Baur, L., Chapman, K., Chapman, S., Gill, T., & King, L. (2014). Digital junk: Food and beverage marketing on facebook. *American Journal of Public Health, 104*(12), e56–e64. https://doi.org/10.2105/AJPH.2014.302167

Gaber, H. R., & Wright, L. T. (2014). Fast-food advertising in social media. A case study on Facebook in Egypt. *Journal of Business and Retail Management Research (JBRMR)* (Vol. 9). Retrieved from www.jbrmr.com

Gensler, S., Völckner, F., Liu-Thompkins, Y., & Wiertz, C. (2013). Managing brands in the social media environment. *Journal of Interactive Marketing, 27*(4), 242–256. https://doi.org/10.1016/j.intmar.2013.09.004

Gortmaker, S. L., Swinburn, B. A., Levy, D., Carter, R., Mabry, P. L., Finegood, D. T., . . . Moodie, M. L. (2011). Changing the future of obesity: Science, policy, and action. *The Lancet, 378*(9793), 838–847. https://doi.org/10.1109/CACS.2014.7097190

Harris, J. L., Brownell, K. D., & Bargh, J. A. (2009). The Food Marketing Defense Model: Integrating psychological research to protect youth and inform public policy. *Social Issues and Policy Review, 3*(1), 211–271. https://doi.org/10.1111/j.1751-2409.2009.01015.x

Harris, J. L., Haraghey, K. S., Lodolce, M., & Semenza, N. L. (2018). Teaching children about good health? Halo effects in child-directed advertisements for unhealthy food. *Pediatric Obesity, 13*(4), 256–264. https://doi.org/10.1111/ijpo.12257

Harris, J. L., Heard, A., & Schwartz, M. (2014). *Older but still vulnerable: All children need protection from unhealthy food marketing.* Retrieved from http://www.uconnruddcenter.org/files/Pdfs/Protecting_Older_Children_3_14.pdf

Harris, J. L., Speers, S. E., Schwartz, M. B., & Brownell, K. D. (2012). US food company branded advergames on the internet: Children's exposure and effects on snack consumption. *Journal of Children and Media, 6*(1), 51–68. https://doi.org/10.1080/17482798.2011.633405

Heath, R. (2009). Emotional engagement: How television builds big brands at low attention. *Journal of Advertising Research, 49*(1), 62–73. https://doi.org/10.2501/S0021849909090060

Heine, C. (2016). Selena Gomez's Social media posts are evidently worth $550,000 apiece – Adweek. Retrieved August 16, 2018, from https://www.adweek.com/digital/selena-gomezs-social-media-posts-are-evidently-worth-550000-apiece-172552/

Henry, H. K. M., & Borzekowski, D. L. G. (2011). The nag factor. *Journal of Children and Media, 5*(3), 298–317. https://doi.org/10.1080/17482798.2011.584380

Hernandez, M. D., & Chapa, S. (2010). Adolescents, advergames and snack foods: Effects of positive affect and experience on memory and choice. *Journal of Marketing Communications, 16*(1–2), 59–68. https://doi.org/10.1080/13527260903342761

Holmberg, C., Chaplin, J., Hillman, T., & Berg, C. (2016). Adolescents' presentation of food in social media: An explorative study. *Appetite, 99*, 121–129. https://doi.org/10.1016/j.appet.2016.01.009

Hsu, H. Y., & Tsou, H.-T. (2011). Understanding customer experiences in online blog environments. *International Journal of Information Management, 31*, 510–523. https://doi.org/10.1016/j.ijinfomgt.2011.05.003

Huang, C. Y., Reisch, L. A., Gwozdz, W., Molnár, D., Konstabel, K., Michels, N., . . . Lissner, L. (2016). Pester power and its consequences: Do European children's food purchasing requests relate to diet and weight outcomes? *Public Health Nutrition.* https://doi.org/10.1017/S136898001600135X

Jenkin, G., Madhvani, N., Signal, L., & Bowers, S. (2014). A systematic review of persuasive marketing techniques to promote food to children on television. *Obesity Reviews, 15*(4), 281–293. https://doi.org/10.1111/obr.12141

Jenkin, G., Signal, L., & Smith, M. (2014). In your face: food marketing to children on Facebook. Retrieved August 23, 2018, from https://foodchildrenandyouth.wordpress.com/

Kelly, B., Bochynska, K., Kornman, K., & Chapman, K. (2008). Internet food marketing on popular children's websites and food product websites in Australia. *Public Health Nutrition, 11*(11), 1180–1187. https://doi.org/10.1017/S1368980008001778

Kelly, B., Freeman, B., King, L., Chapman, K., Baur, L. A., & Gill, T. (2016). Television advertising, not viewing, is associated with negative dietary patterns in children. *Pediatric Obesity, 11*(2), 158–160. https://doi.org/10.1111/ijpo.12057

Kelly, B., Halford, J. C. G., Boyland, E. J., Chapman, K., Bautista-Castaño, I., Berg, C., . . . Summerbell, C. (2010). Television food advertising to children: A global perspective. *American Journal of Public Health, 100*(9), 1730–1736. https://doi.org/10.2105/AJPH.2009.179267

Kelly, B., King, L., Chapman, K., Boyland, E., Bauman, A. E., & Baur, L. A. (2015). A hierarchy of unhealthy food promotion effects: Identifying methodological approaches and knowledge gaps. *American Journal of Public Health, 105*(4), e86–e95. https://doi.org/10.2105/AJPH.2014.302476

Kelly, B., Vandevijvere, S., Freeman, B., & Jenkin, G. (2015). New media but same old tricks: Food marketing to children in the digital age. *Current Obesity Reports, 4*(1), 37–45. https://doi.org/10.1007/s13679-014-0128-5

Kent, M. P., & Pauzé, E. (2018). The effectiveness of self-regulation in limiting the advertising of unhealthy foods and beverages on children's preferred websites in Canada. *Public Health Nutrition, 21*(9), 1608–1617. https://doi.org/10.1017/S1368980017004177

Kim, A. J., & Johnson, K. K. P. (2016). Power of consumers using social media: Examining the influences of brand-related user-generated content on Facebook. *Computers in Human Behavior, 58*, 98–108. https://doi.org/10.1016/j.chb.2015.12.047

Knoll, J., & Matthes, J. (2017). The effectiveness of celebrity endorsements: A meta-analysis. *Journal of the Academy of Marketing Science, 45*(1), 55–75. https://doi.org/10.1007/s11747-016-0503-8

Kunkel, D. (2001). Children and television advertising. In D. Singer & J. Singer (Eds.), *Handbook of children and the media.* (pp. 375–393). Thousand Oaks, CA: Sage.

Lake, A., & Townsend, T. (2006). Obesogenic environments: exploring the built and food environments. *The Journal of The Royal Society for the Promotion of Health, 126*(6), 262–267.

Lawlor, M.-A., Dunne, Á., & Rowley, J. (2016). Young consumers' brand communications literacy in a social networking site context. *European Journal of Marketing, 50*(11), 2018–2040. https://doi.org/http://dx.doi.org/10.1108/MRR-09-2015-0216

Linn, S. E. (2013). Food marketing to children in the context of a marketing maelstrom. *Journal of Public Health Policy, 25*(3), 367–378.

Lobstein, T., & Dibb, S. (2005). Evidence of a possible link between obesogenic food advertising and child overweight. *Obesity Reviews.* https://doi.org/10.1111/j.1467-789X.2005.00191.x

Mallinckrodt, V., & Mizerski, D. (2007). The effects of playing an advergame on young children's perceptions, preferences, and requests. *Journal of Advertising, 36*(2), 87–100. https://doi.org/10.2753/JOA0091-3367360206

McDermott, L., O'Sullivan, T., Stead, M., & Hastings. (2006). International food advertising, pester power and its effects. *International Journal of Advertising.* https://doi.org/10.1080/02650487.2006.11072986

McGuire, W. (1976). Some internal psychological factors influencing consumer choice. *Journal of Consumer Research, 2*(4), 302–319.

Mendoza, L. (2015). *Persuading teens to ' Share a Coke .'* Retrieved from https://www.mrs.org.uk/pdf/US_COCA_COLA_-_FINAL_TWO.pdf

Montgomery, K. C. (2015). Youth and surveillance in the Facebook era: Policy interventions and social implications. *Telecommunications Policy, 39*, 771–786. https://doi.org/10.1016/j.telpol.2014.12.006

Ng, S. H., Kelly, B., Se, C. H., Chinna, K., Sameeha, J., Krishnasamy, S., . . . Sameeha, M. J. (2014). Global health action obesogenic television food advertising to children in Malaysia: Sociocultural variations. *Global Health Action, 7*(1), 25169. https://doi.org/10.3402/gha.v7.25169org/10.3402/gha.v7.25169

Norman, J., Kelly, B., McMahon, A. T., Boyland, E., Baur, L. A., Chapman, K., . . . Bauman, A. (2018). Sustained impact of energy-dense TV and online food advertising on children's dietary intake: A within-subject, randomised, crossover, counter-balanced trial. *International Journal of Behavioral Nutrition and Physical Activity, 15*(1). https://doi.org/10.1186/s12966-018-0672-6

Obesity Health Alliance. (2017). *A "watershed" moment. Why it's prime time to protect children from junk food adverts.* Retrieved from http://obesityhealthalliance.org.uk/wp-content/uploads/2017/11/A-Watershed-Moment-report.pdf

Ofcom. (2016). Children and parents: Media use and attitudes report, 1–53. Retrieved from https://www.ofcom.org.uk/__data/assets/pdf_file/0034/93976/Children-Parents-Media-Use-Attitudes-Report-2016.pdf

Owen, L., Lewis, C., Auty, S., & Buijzen, M. (2013). Is children's understanding of nontraditional advertising comparable to their understanding of television advertising? *Journal of Public Policy & Marketing, 32*(2), 195–206. https://doi.org/10.1509/jppm.09.003

Pettigrew, S., Rosenberg, M., Ferguson, R., Houghton, S., & Wood, L. (2013). Game on: Do children absorb sports sponsorship messages? *Public Health Nutrition, 16*(12), 2197–2204. https://doi.org/10.1017/S1368980012005435

Powell, L. M., Schermbeck, R. M., & Chaloupka, F. J. (2013). Nutritional content of food and beverage products in television advertisements seen on children's programming. *Childhood Obesity, 9*(6), 524–531. https://doi.org/10.1089/chi.2013.0072

Reidenberg, J. R., Breaux, T., Cranor, L. F., & French, B. M. (2015). *Disagreeable privacy policies: Mismatches between meaning and users' understanding, 30 Berkeley Tech. L. J* (Vol. 39). Retrieved from http://ir.lawnet.fordham.edu/faculty_scholarshipAvailableat:http://ir.lawnet.fordham.edu/faculty_scholarship/619Electroniccopyavailableat:http://ssrn.com/abstract=2418297Electroniccopyavailableat:http://ssrn.com/abstract=2418297

Richardson, J., & Harris, J. L. (2011). *Food marketing and social media: Findings from Fast Food FACTS and Sugary Drink FACTS.* Retrieved from http://www.uconnruddcenter.org/files/Pdfs/FoodMarketingSocialMedia_AmericanUniversity_11_11.pdf

Robinson, T. N., Borzekowski, D. L. G., Matheson, D. M., & Kraemer, H. C. (2007). Effects of fast food branding on young children's taste preferences. *Archives of Pediatrics & Adolescent Medicine, 161*(8), 792. https://doi.org/10.1001/archpedi.161.8.792

Royo-Bordonada, M., León-Flández, K., Damián, J., Bosqued-Estefanía, M. J., Moya-Geromini, M., & López-Jurado, L. (2016). The extent and nature of food advertising to children on Spanish television in 2012 using an international food-based coding system and the UK nutrient profiling model. *Public Health, 137,* 88–94. https://doi.org/10.1016/j.puhe.2016.03.001

Rozendaal, E., Lapierre, M. A., van Reijmersdal, E. A., & Buijzen, M. (2011). Reconsidering advertising literacy as a defense against advertising effects. *Media Psychology, 14*(4), 333–354. https://doi.org/10.1080/15213269.2011.620540

Russell, S. J., Croker, H., & Viner, R. M. (2018). The effect of screen advertising on children's dietary intake: A systematic review and meta-analysis. *Obesity Reviews* (August), 1–15. https://doi.org/10.1111/obr.12812

Sadeghirad, B., Duhaney, T., Motaghipisheh, S., Campbell, N. R. C., & Johnston, B. C. (2016). Influence of unhealthy food and beverage marketing on children's dietary intake and preference: A systematic review and meta-analysis of randomized trials. *Obesity Reviews, 17*(10), 945–959. https://doi.org/10.1111/obr.12445

Schor, J. B., & Ford, M. (2007). From taste great to cool: Children' s food marketing and the rise of the symbolic. *Journal of Law, Medicine & Ethics*, 10–21. Retrieved from https:// content.ebscohost.com/ContentServer.asp?T=P&P=AN&K=502558087&S=R&D=lf t&EbscoContent=dGJyMMTo50SeprU40dvuOLCmr1CeprJSsqi4SreWxWXS&Conte ntCustomer=dGJyMOzprkmvqLJPuePfgeyx44Dt6flA

Smits, T., Vandebosch, H., Neyens, E., & Boyland, E. (2015). The persuasiveness of child-targeted endorsement strategies: A systematic review. *Annals of the International Communication Association*, *39*(1), 311–337. https://doi.org/10.1080/23808985.2015.1 1679179

Statistica.com. (2018). Children and media in the U.S. Retrieved August 9, 2018, from https://www.statista.com/topics/3980/children-and-media-in-the-us/

Stevenson, D. (2014). *Data and discrimination: Collected essays*. Retrieved from https:// s3.amazonaws.com/www.newamerica.org/downloads/OTI-Data-an-Discrimination-FINAL-small.pdf

Story, M., & French, S. (2004). Food advertising and marketing directed at children and adolescents in the US. *International Journal of Behavioral Nutrition and Physical Activity*, *1*, 3. https://doi.org/10.1186/1479-5868-1-3

Sütterlin, B., & Siegrist, M. (2015). Simply adding the word "fruit" makes sugar healthier: The misleading effect of symbolic information on the perceived healthiness of food. *Appetite*. https://doi.org/10.1016/j.appet.2015.07.011

Swinburn, B. A., Sacks, G., Hall, K. D., Mcpherson, K., Finegood, D. T., Moodie, M. L., & Gortmaker, S. L. (2011). Obesity 1 The global obesity pandemic: shaped by global drivers and local environments. *The Lancet*, *378*, 804–814. https://doi.org/10.1016/ S0140-6736(11)60813-1

Tan, L., See Hoe, N., Azahadi, O., & Tilakavati, K. (2018). What's on YouTube? A case study on food and beverage advertising in videos targeted at children on social media. *Chlldhood Obesity*, *14*(4), 280–290. https://doi.org/10.1089/chi.2018.0037

Tatlow-Golden, M., Tracey, L., & Dolphin, L. (2016). *Irish Heart Foundation. Who's feeding the kids online?* Retrieved from www.irishheart.ie

The Drum. (2018). Teens, YouTube and the rise of the micro-influencers. Retrieved August 17, 2018, from https://www.thedrum.com/opinion/2018/06/26/teens-you-tube-and-the-rise-the-micro-influencers

Turow, J. (2011). Targets or waste. In *The daily you: How the new advertising industry is defining your identity and your worth* (pp. 88–110). New Haven: Yale University Press.

Van Den Berg, S. W., Boer, J. M., Scholtens, S., De Jongste, J. C., Brunekreef, B., Smit, H. A., & Wijga, A. H. (2011). Quantification of the energy gap in young over-weight children. the PIAMA birth cohort study. *BMC Public Health*, *11*. https://doi. org/10.1186/1471-2458-11-326

Vassallo, A. J., Kelly, B., Zhang, L., Wang, Z., Young, S., & Freeman, B. (2018). Junk Food marketing on Instagram: Content analysis. *JMIR Public Health and Surveillance*, *4*(2), e54. https://doi.org/10.2196/publichealth.9594

Wang, Y., & Lim, H. (2012). The global childhood obesity epidemic and the association between socio-economic status and childhood obesity. *International Review of Psychiatry*, *24*(3), 176–188. https://doi.org/10.3109/09540261.2012.688195

Whalen, R., Harrold, J., Child, S., Halford, J., & Boyland, E. (2017). Children's exposure to food advertising: The impact of statutory restrictions. *Health Promotion International*. https://doi.org/10.1093/heapro/dax044

Whalen, R., Harrold, J., Child, S., Halford, J., & Boyland, E. (2018). The health halo trend in UK television food advertising viewed by children: The rise of implicit and explicit health messaging in the promotion of unhealthy foods. *International Journal of Environmental Research and Public Health*, *15*(3), 560. https://doi.org/10.3390/ijerph15030560

WHO. (2010). *Set of recommendations on the marketing of foods and non-alcoholic beverages to children*. Geneva: WHO. Retrieved from http://apps.who.int/iris/bitstream/handle/10665/44416/9789241500210_eng.pdf;jsessionid=020E3A91BA6F288A69D3A9554F1926D9?sequence=1

WHO. (2013). *Marketing of foods high in fat, salt and sugar to children. Update 2012–2013.* Copenhagen: WHO.

WHO. (2016). *Tackling food marketing to children in a digital world: Trans-disciplinary perspectives.* Retrieved from http://www.euro.who.int/__data/assets/pdf_file/0017/322226/Tackling-food-marketing-children-digital-world-trans-disciplinary-perspectives-en.pdf

WHO. (2018). *Evaluating implementation of the WHO set of challenges and guidance for next steps in the WHO non-alcoholic beverages to children*: Retrieved from http://www.euro.who.int/pubrequest

Wright, P., Friestad, M., & Boush, D. M. (2005). The development of marketplace persuasion knowledge in children, adolescents, and young adults. *Journal of Public Policy & Marketing*, *24*(2), 222–223.

2

FOOD MARKETING TO ADOLESCENTS AND YOUNG ADULTS

Skeptical but still under the influence

Dr. Jennifer L. Harris and Dr. Frances Fleming-Milici

Food marketing and its impact on skyrocketing rates of obesity have become a worldwide public health crisis. Food advertising to children and adolescents almost exclusively promotes high-fat, sugar, and sodium (HFSS) food and drinks, and it increases their preferences and requests to parents for unhealthy products (Hastings et al., 2003; Institute of Medicine [IOM], 2006; World Health Organization [WHO], 2010). Food advertising also increases children's consumption of any available food (Boyland et al. 2016; Harris, Bargh, & Brownell, 2009) and highly advertised product categories (e.g., soda and fast food) (Andreyeva, Kelly, & Harris, 2011).

In response to public health concerns, the food industry has enacted voluntary self-regulatory initiatives to limit unhealthy advertising to children (Hawkes, 2007). A small number of countries have also enacted food marketing legislation (WHO, 2012). However, most of these policies only address advertising to children under age 12 or 13 (WHO, 2012).

This focus on young children is based on extensive psychological research demonstrating children's limited understanding of persuasive intent until age 11 or 12 (IOM, 2006). Yet relatively few studies have examined effects of marketing on adolescents or young adults (ages 13–24), thus limiting any conclusions regarding effects on youth older than age 12. Furthermore, existing policies assume that adolescents' cognitive abilities to recognize persuasive intent and express skepticism about advertising enable them to defend against unwanted influence (Boush, Friestadt, & Rose, 1994). However, these abilities do not necessarily protect adolescents or even adults from harmful effects of HFSS food marketing (Harris, Brownell & Bargh, 2009). In addition, understanding of persuasive intent in newer, often disguised, forms of marketing has not been well investigated, and processing of these messages differs significantly from traditional marketing messages (Buijzen, Van Reijmersdal, & Owen, 2010).

In this chapter, we present evidence that knowledge of persuasive intent is not sufficient and that food marketing also contributes to diet-related health risks among adolescents and young adults. We first describe food marketing to these age groups, including highly promoted product categories and the variety of marketing techniques used. Second, we discuss the psychological mechanisms through which marketing influences all consumers, often outside of their awareness, and present the conditions that are necessary to defend against food marketing effects effectively. Third, we present unique developmental processes that make adolescents and young adults especially vulnerable to influence. Finally, we summarize research needed to inform potential solutions that effectively address unhealthy food marketing to adolescents and young adults.

The food marketing environment

Massive investments in HFSS food marketing have fueled the obesity crisis (IOM, 2006; WHO, 2010). US food, beverage, and restaurant companies spent $13.4 billion on advertising in all media in 2017 (Harris, Frazier, Kumanyika, & Ramirez, 2019), and this marketing often targets adolescents (ages 12–17), as well as children under 12 (U.S. Federal Trade Commission [FTC], 2012).

Despite years of public health appeals to market healthy food, the vast majority of this marketing continues to promote unhealthy food and drinks (Cairns, Angus, Hastings, & Caraher, 2013; Harris et al., 2017). Calorie-dense HFSS product categories, including fast-food restaurants, candy, sugar-sweetened beverages (SSBs), and savory and sweet snacks, represented 70% of US TV food advertising spending in 2017 (Harris, Frazier, Kumanyika, et al., 2019). In contrast, healthier product categories (including 100% juice, plain water, nuts, and fruits and vegetables) represented just 3% of advertising.

The majority of adolescent-targeted food marketing also promotes fast food, SSBs, sugary cereals, snacks, and sweets (FTC, 2012). Research has not documented the extent of food marketing to young adults, but millennials (i.e., ages 18–34) represent a highly desirable market due to their purchasing power and high engagement with multiple forms of media (Nielsen, 2017). This demographic group, especially young males, represents a key advertising segment for fast-food and SSB companies (Nelson, Story, Larson, Neumark-Sztainer, & Lytle, 2008). The billions that companies invest in marketing to adolescents and young adults demonstrate that it must be highly effective at generating purchases and consumption of fast food, SSBs, candy, snacks, and other highly advertised products.

Newer forms of food marketing

Food companies continue to spend the majority of their advertising budgets on television (Harris, Frazier, Kumanyika, et al., 2019). However, commercial TV viewing is declining, especially among adolescents and young adults (Friedman, 2017). Millennials also watch less TV than older adults (Statista, 2019b). Although the majority of food marketing research has focused on TV advertising (IOM, 2006), food companies also invest heavily in other forms of marketing to reach adolescents, including digital marketing, sponsorships (of events, athletics, and philanthropies), marketing in schools, and in-store marketing and packaging (FTC, 2012).

Evolving digital marketing

According to the FTC (2012), digital marketing (i.e., marketing on digital devices, including PCs and smartphones) represented just 6.9% of total youth-directed food marketing expenditures in 2009, but teen-targeted digital marketing expenditures increased by 51% from 2006 to 2009. These data have not been updated since 2009; however, digital marketing has likely increased in importance as smartphone usage among adolescents and young adults has ballooned since then. Ninety-five percent of teens report having a smartphone or having access to one, and nearly one-half (45%) report being online "almost constantly" (Anderson & Jiang, 2018). Time spent on social media is also increasing. In 2016, 82% of 12th-graders said they visited social media sites "almost every day" (Twenge, Martin, & Spitzberg, 2018). To keep up with changing media usage patterns, food companies have also been early adopters of newer forms of marketing in digital media to reach adolescents and young adults (Statista, 2019a).

Social media marketing, or the practice of using social media platforms (e.g., Facebook, Instagram, YouTube, Twitter) to promote a brand, is one of the most common forms of digital food marketing. Social media sites have become the most widely used websites for food companies to post their online advertising (Harris et al., 2017). The majority of highly advertised US food brands also maintain accounts on social media platforms that are popular with young people (Harris et al., 2017). These accounts include company-generated posts designed to encourage brand engagement, such as contents, games, quizzes, and apps, as well as user-generated content in the form of comments and other information posted by users. On YouTube, food brands maintain their own channels where viewers can access commercials and share them virally with their friends. Fast food (Harris et al., 2013), SSB (Harris et al., 2014), and snack food brands (Harris et al., 2015) rank among the top brands on social media, with the most active brands posting hundreds of times per day.

Social media influencers are also extremely popular with adolescents and young adults, and influencers have become a common marketing tool for food companies to reach youth. Brands pay these celebrities, monetarily and/or by receiving free products, to endorse products in their blogs and social media posts (Freberg, Graham, McGaughey, & Freberg, 2011). Influencers include traditional celebrities (e.g., musicians, athletes, actors) and celebrities created solely by their digital presence. Online influencers differ from traditional celebrities as they engage directly with consumers through their social media accounts, a process termed "parasocial interaction," and they embed promotion of brands into personal stories they share online (Lueck, 2015).

Food companies also market through mobile apps, which individuals download to their smartphones (Montgomery, Grier, Chester, & Dorfman, 2013). Fast-food and SSB brands were among the first to offer branded mobile apps for users to place orders, receive coupons and offers, play branded games, and/or post on social media (Harris et al., 2013, 2014). Mobile apps raise numerous privacy and other concerns as they allow companies to access users' contacts and other information stored on their devices. Companies also utilize phones' GPS capabilities to send offers and other advertising content in or near the point of sale, encouraging impulse purchases.

Youth exposure to newer forms of digital marketing is more difficult for academic researchers to measure as companies own these data and they are not publicly available. Furthermore, exposure is highly individualized, due to companies' viral distribution and proprietary algorithms. However, these tactics likely allow food companies to reach large numbers of adolescents and young adults. In an analysis of the most popular food and beverage Facebook pages in Australia, nearly all appealed most to adolescents (ages 13–17) and/or young adults (ages 18–24) (Freeman et al., 2014). In a US study of adolescents, 70% reported that they liked, shared, or followed at least one food or beverage brand on social media (Fleming-Milici & Harris, 2019). They engaged with six brands on average, while approximately one-third reported engaging with five or more brands. Fast food, sugary drinks, snacks, and candy brands were most popular.

Other marketing techniques

As noted earlier, companies also frequently target adolescents with marketing outside of media, including sponsorships and retail-based promotions. Teen-targeted food company expenditures on some of these types of marketing increased from 2006 to 2009, including celebrity endorsements (+98%), sponsorships (+17%), and premiums (+11%) (FTC, 2012). These forms of marketing are also difficult to track as they typically vary by location and may occur for a short time, so they have received considerably less research attention. However, a few US studies have examined the extent of food brand product placements in TV and movies, sports sponsorships, and celebrity endorsements.

Two-thirds of product placements in movies that were popular with children, adolescents, and young adults contained at least one food or beverage brand (Sutherland, MacKenzie, Purvis, & Dalton, 2010). Three-quarters of beverage placements were for SSBs, while candy and salty snacks represented almost one-half of food placements. On prime-time TV, US adolescents viewed as many as 110 food and beverage brand placements in one year, consisting primarily of SSB and fast-food brands (Elsey & Harris, 2016). SSB placements on reality TV talent competitions attracted the most teen viewers. Notably, these placements lasted up to 60 seconds, including branded cups sitting on judges' desks and sponsored vignettes about contestants.

Another study examined the ten sports organizations with the highest youth (under age 18) TV audience and identified 44 food and non-alcoholic beverage sponsors, exceeded only by automotive sponsors (Bragg et al., 2018). Soft drinks and sports drinks represented three-quarters of beverage sponsorships, while three-quarters of food sponsorships were for snack foods, candy, and fast food. Similarly, music celebrities popular with teens endorsed more than 100 food and non-alcoholic beverage brands, most frequently full-calorie soft drinks (Bragg, Miller, Elizee, Dighe, & Elbel, 2016); endorsements also included energy drink, fast food, and snack brands.

Psychology of food marketing effects

As noted, research on food marketing effects has focused on children's understanding of persuasive intent and assumes that this understanding leads to the ability to defend against undesirable marketing attempts. This information-processing approach to persuasion (McGuire, 1976) posits a sequential path from marketing exposure to consumer behavior. According to this model, consumers attend to and actively process information presented in marketing before making a conscious rational decision about product purchases and/or consumption.

Research on consumer development has found that children possess the cognitive ability to activate their knowledge of advertising tactics to defend against advertising exposure by age 12–14 (John, 1999). By age 11 or 12 children are highly skeptical of advertising, expressing disbelief about advertising claims and mistrust of advertisers' motives (Boush et al., 1994). Through early adolescence, knowledge about advertising tactics increases. According to the information-processing approach, when an individual can recognize that a message is marketing and has the cognitive ability to consider the information and make an informed decision, then s/he can defend against persuasive attempts.

However, some researchers have questioned this assumption (Harris, Brownell, et al., 2009; Rozendaal, Lapierre, Buijzen, & Van Reijmersdal, 2011). Despite high levels of skepticism, adolescents express significant enjoyment and engagement with advertising (Moore & Lutz, 2000). Furthermore, skepticism about advertising does not necessarily reduce preferences for advertised products (e.g., Chernin, 2008). Therefore, the ability to understand persuasive intent may be necessary, but not sufficient to adequately defend against food marketing effects among adolescents or young adults.

Emotional marketing

One explanation for how marketing influences attitudes and behaviors despite expressed skepticism about advertising is that marketing effects often occur on an emotional level, effectively bypassing a rational information-processing response. An examination of 880 different advertising campaigns found that campaigns with emotional messages had stronger business effects (e.g., higher sales, increased brand preferences) than those with rational messages (Binet & Field, 2009). The authors concluded that "*The most effective advertisements of all are those with little or no rational content*" (p. 131). Marketers distinguish between "informational" and "emotional" marketing messages (Advertising Research Foundation, 2008). In the case of food marketing, where the goal is to brand commodity products with few tangible differences, nearly all messages are emotional. Consider the Coca-Cola polar bears or McDonald's images of family bonding over a Happy Meal. These emotional messages are designed to distinguish Coca-Cola from other colas, and McDonald's from other fast-food restaurants.

Marketing researchers have adopted cognitive psychology to describe brand attitudes, including emotional connections to brands, as networks of associations. In these "brand schemas," the brand name/logo is the central node linked to all other concepts experienced together with the brand (including emotions, usage occasions, other users, product attributes) (Keller, 2003). According to the theory of spreading activation, when consumers encounter a brand or any linked concept, this schema automatically activates and strengthens over time (Keller, 2003).

Therefore, exposure to marketing creates brand associations and strengthens the brand relationship with every exposure (Heath, 2000). Successful marketers devise advertising linking their brands with core human motivations (e.g., accomplishment, belonging, self-fulfillment) (Wansink, 2003) and ensure that every marketing message reinforces these associations, including packaging, retail locations, sponsorships, and influencers, as well advertising. Two food brands popular with US teens epitomize this approach: Gatorade advertising features motivational Black athlete celebrities and sports science to appeal to aspiring athletes (Akopyan, 2017), while Doritos packaging and advertising convey a bold and daring image that resonates with adolescents and young adults (Mohan, 2013). Upon repeated exposure to attractive marketing stimuli paired with food brands, these positive associations create positive brand images, brand preferences, and consumption, through a psychological process called "affective conditioning." Furthermore, affective conditioning occurs even in the absence of positive stimuli due to the "mere exposure effect" (Monahan, Murphy, & Zajonc, 2000). Incidental exposure to brand names and/or logos alone can increase positive brand attitudes and choice (Ferraro, Bettman, & Chartrand, 2008; Janiszewski, 1993).

According to schema theory, exposure to marketing can also affect behavior directly by priming automatic associations with those behaviors. Exposure to food advertising leads children to consume more of any available food, not just foods presented in the ads (Boyland et al., 2016). Furthermore, these effects occur automatically, outside of conscious awareness, and they have been shown with young adults as well as children (Harris, Bargh, et al., 2009). When questioned to assess awareness of the research purpose, participants were not aware that their exposure to food advertising might have affected their eating behavior.

Resisting food marketing influence

Understanding how food marketing may affect individuals automatically, outside of conscious awareness, also provides insights into the difficulties of resisting advertising effects, even for mature adults who have the cognitive ability to do so. According to the Persuasion Knowledge Model, recognition of persuasive intent is necessary but not sufficient to defend against advertising (Friestad & Wright, 1994). Experience is also required to learn how to effectively defend against different types of advertising, which develops throughout life with exposure to different types of persuasive attempts. For adults, the best predictor of negative attitudes about advertising occurs when individuals actively counterargue the messages in the ad (Wright, 1973). Therefore, according to the Persuasion Knowledge Model, because individuals are less aware of emotional effects and other automatic responses to advertising, these types of persuasive messages will be more effective than direct arguments about product benefits.

These automatic food marketing effects represent a form of "mental contamination" from external stimuli. According to Wilson and Brekke (1994), several conditions are necessary to defend against these unwanted effects: the cognitive ability to resist; awareness of how one is influenced by the stimuli; and the motivation to resist. The Food Marketing Defense Model (FMDM) adapts this model to food marketing effects (Harris, Brownell, et al., 2009). FMDM (Box 2.1) proposes four necessary conditions to defend against influence of unhealthy food marketing: (1) *awareness* of marketing stimuli, including conscious attention to a stimulus and understanding of its persuasive intent; (2) *understanding* of how one is affected and the outcome (e.g., liking the brand, consuming more food) and understanding how to resist that influence effectively; (3) *cognitive ability* to resist, as well as available cognitive resources at the time of exposure; and (4) *motivation* to resist.

BOX 2.1   THE FOOD MARKETING DEFENSE MODEL (FMDM)*

Necessary conditions to defend against food marketing influence effectively

Awareness

- Attend to marketing stimuli
- Comprehend persuasive intent

Understanding

- Understand underlying processes and outcomes
- Understand how to resist effectively

Ability

- Cognitive ability to resist effectively
- Available cognitive resources

Motivation

- Interest and desire to resist

*From Harris, Brownell, and Bargh (2009).

Considering the effects of marketing through this theoretical framework provides insights into how marketing influences adolescents and adults, despite their
understanding of persuasive intent and skepticism of marketing. This framework
also explains how marketing can bypass conscious information processing and affect
brand attitudes and behaviors automatically, and why effective emotional advertising is so powerful. Watching an ad that activates an emotional response will distract
from considering the information (or lack of it) in the ad, thus deactivating a skeptical
response. Therefore, ad liking is one of the strongest predictors of brand liking in
children and adults (Moore & Lutz, 2000). This process can also explain how hidden
forms of marketing, such as product placements embedded in movies, TV programming, games, and music, and "influencer" marketing, can increase brand preferences,
even when the viewer does not notice the brand message (Eisenberg, McDowell,
Berestein, Tsiantar, & Finan, 2002).

Developmental vulnerabilities

Although advertising may be more efficient at creating brand schemas in younger
children whose brains are rapidly developing, brain development occurs across
the lifespan. In addition, adolescents' still-developing cognitive abilities to delay
gratification, increasing independence, and the means to purchase their own food
may make them uniquely vulnerable to the influence of unhealthy food marketing.
For these reasons, public health experts have called on food companies to expand
the food industry self-regulation to cover adolescents up through at least 14 years
old (Healthy Eating Research, 2015). However, many of these developmental vulnerabilities continue through early adulthood (Dietz, 2017; Nelson et al., 2008).
Life transitions, such as living independently for the first time, working full-time,
marrying, and having children, present opportunities, as well as risks, for adopting behaviors that promote health and prevent disease during young adulthood
(Nelson et al., 2008). Health behavior patterns established during this lifestage
predict weight gain and lifetime chronic disease risk, including obesity, type 2
diabetes, hypertension, and cardiovascular disease (Dietz, 2017).

As noted, food marketers commonly target adolescents and young adults with
marketing for their least nutritious products. In addition, companies commonly
use marketing techniques that hide their persuasive intent to deactivate skeptical
responses and also take advantage of young people's unique developmental vulnerabilities, reducing their motivation to resist influence.

Worsening dietary patterns

With increasing independence and responsibility for their own food choices, dietary patterns worsen during adolescence and young adulthood, resulting in weight
gain and increasing rates of obesity (Dietz, 2017; Nelson et al., 2008). Adolescents
and young adults are also the most frequent consumers of many highly advertised
products, including fast food, sugary drinks, and HFSS snacks, that contribute to
weight gain (Harris, Frazier, Kumanyika, et al., 2019, Nelson et al., 2008).

Almost 40% of calories consumed by adolescents (ages 12–18) are empty calories in the form of added sugar and solid fats (almost 800 calories per day), and almost one-half of these calories come from SSBs, desserts, and pizza (Reedy & Krebs-Smith, 2010). On average, SSBs represent 10% of calories consumed by adolescents (225 calories per day), compared to 6–7% of calories for children and adults (Bleich, Vercammen, Koma, & Li, 2018). Further, US adolescents and young adults consume more salty snacks and candy than any other age group (Rudd Center, 2013). On a given day, 41% of teens consume fast food, resulting in 310 additional calories (Powell, Nguyen, & Han, 2012). Young adults are the most frequent consumers of fast food, with more than one-half of 20–39-year-olds reporting that they ate fast food on a given day (Paeratakul, Ferdinand, Champagne, Ryan, & Bray, 2003).

Together with worsening dietary habits, obesity prevalence increases during this time, from 17% for children (6–11 years) and 21% for adolescents (12–19 years), to 34% among adults (20–39 years) (Flegal, Kruszon-Moran, Carroll, Fryar, & Ogden, 2016; Ogden et al., 2016). SSB consumption is positively associated with obesity rates among children and adults (Luger et al., 2017). Fast food consumption in adolescence also predicts weight gain from adolescence to adulthood (Niemeier, Raynor, Lloyd-Richardson, Rogers, & Wing, 2006).

Awareness

Many newer forms of marketing targeting adolescents and young adults, including social media, product placements, and sponsorships, appear to be designed to hide their persuasive intent and reduce awareness that they are marketing stimuli, thus deactivating skeptical responses. If an individual is not aware of the persuasive intent of the message, or the message does not activate a skeptical response for another reason, then the message recipient cannot defend against the persuasive attempt (Friestad & Wright, 1994; Harris, Brownell, et al., 2009). These "stealth marketing" tactics may be unfair and deceptive, raising ethical issues (Petty & Andrews, 2008).

Furthermore, hidden forms of marketing may be even more difficult to resist than TV advertising (Friestad & Wright, 1994; Harris, Brownell, et al., 2009). Marketing embedded within entertainment or other content (e.g., product placements in TV and movies, social media and blog posts, YouTube commercial videos, sponsorships) is less recognizable as marketing. Only 62% of 12–15-year-olds who go online were aware that video bloggers might be paid to endorse brands, and less than one-third identified paid search results as ads, even when the result was outlined in an orange box and labeled with the word "Ad" (OFCOM, 2017). In some cases, individuals may not see the commercial messages at all, as in product placements in the background of movies and TV programming.

"Advertising disclosure" statements have been proposed to increase awareness of hidden marketing, but they may not reduce its effectiveness. One study found that disclosures during brand placements in TV programming increased adolescents' and adults' ability to recognize the placements as marketing, but it did not reduce the persuasive effect (Van Reijmersdal, Boerman, Rozendaal, & Buijzen, 2017). Furthermore, the disclosure increased memory of the brand for adolescents. In a study of energy drink social media content, adolescents and young adults understood that the messages were designed to promote energy drinks, but they valued the companies' "honesty" in disclosing the ingredients in the drinks and their corporate social responsibility in supporting contributions to charities and environmental efforts (Buchanan, Kelly, & Yeatman, 2017). Engagement with entertainment content, such as in branded games and sponsorships, also may distract the user from the persuasive intent of these marketing messages and deactivate skeptical responses.

Social media posts shared virally through peer networks come disguised as messages from friends, representing another hidden form of marketing (Dunlop, Freeman, & Jones, 2016; Montgomery et al., 2013). Brand posts on social media appear to be generated by peers and not the company, which may increase their effectiveness versus traditional brand-generated forms of marketing (Soneji et al., 2018). Furthermore, exposure to positive user-generated content on brands' Facebook accounts was associated with emotional and cognitive responses, which led to increased brand engagement and future purchase intent (Kim & Johnson, 2016). A qualitative analysis of young adults' responses to energy drink social media content indicated that posts from other users had more influence on participants' attitudes toward and intent to purchase and consume energy drinks than brand-generated posts (Buchanan et al., 2017).

Cognitive ability

The FMDM also posits that still-developing executive control abilities during adolescence and young adulthood also increase their vulnerability to influence from unhealthy food marketing. These vulnerabilities have not been well studied in the food marketing literature. However, alcohol and tobacco advertising researchers have demonstrated that adolescents are more susceptible to marketing influence than adults due to greater impulsivity and increased reward sensitivity (Pechmann, Levine, Loughlin, & Leslie, 2005), and similar processes likely affect adolescents' responses to food marketing.

Most adolescents know what behaviors are in their best long-term interest (e.g., eating healthily), but the executive control required to resist immediate gratification (e.g., a tempting snack or SSB) to achieve a long-term goal (e.g., good health) does not fully develop until their mid-20s (Arain et al., 2013). Hormones and brain development also heighten reward sensitivity during adolescence (Galvan, 2013). Furthermore, decision making and impulse control become more difficult for adolescents when emotional arousal and/or resisting peer influence are involved, increasing their risk of making poor choices (Albert, Chein, & Steinberg, 2013). Therefore, adolescents may be more susceptible to emotional advertising and advertising for unhealthy, but highly rewarding, products, compared to adults and perhaps even younger children.

A few studies examining adolescents' neural responses during exposure to food marketing support this hypothesis. One functional magnetic resonance imaging study showed greater attention and reward responsivity to TV food advertisements compared to other TV ads among adolescents (ages 14–17) (Gearhardt, Yokum, Stice, Harris, & Brownell, 2014). Reward responsivity was not associated with body mass index in that study, but it predicted weight gain 1 year later (Yokum, Gearhardt, Harris, Brownell, & Stice, 2014). Additional studies have shown similar neural responses to Coca-Cola advertisements in adolescents (Burger & Stice, 2014), and to food logos alone (Bruce et al., 2014).

Motivation

Adolescents' psychological development also likely reduces their motivation to resist unhealthy food marketing by taking advantage of heightened peer influence and their need to establish their own identities. From childhood through early adolescence, concern about peers increases whereas parental influence on consumer behaviors declines (Dotson & Hyatt, 2005). Young adolescents are highly susceptible to information about what is "cool" or "in" conveyed through advertising (Valkenburg & Cantor, 2001). Concerns about peers peak by age 14 (Steinberg & Monahan, 2007), which makes younger adolescents especially susceptible to marketing messages shared by peers, such as viral videos or social media posts.

Adolescents also use brands to help create their own identities, increasing their susceptibility to advertising that portrays popularity and status from consuming food brands (Pechmann et al., 2005). For example, positive brand images in soft drink ads increased adolescents' ratings of the ads, brands, and products (Kelly, Slater, & Karan, 2002), while both children and adolescents rated unhealthy brands as more cool, fun, and exciting and their users as more popular, compared to healthier brands (Kelly et al., 2016). Furthermore, participants perceived that other children would want to make friends with the personified unhealthier brands than with the healthier brands. In focus groups with low-income Black and Latino adolescents, participants readily discussed their perceptions of people who consume different food brands and appeared to internalize brand images for some popular brands (Harris, Frazier, Fleming-Milici, et al., 2019). For example, they discussed how Doritos' commercials (described earlier) created an image that Doritos consumers are popular and fun, while Gatorade commercials were especially motivational for aspiring young male athletes.

Some marketing increases young people's identification with brands, which can also reduce their motivation to resist influence. For example, adolescents who expressed stronger connections with television characters were more affected by TV product placements (Russell, Norman, & Heckler, 2004). Similarly, users who engage with online influencers feel they know and trust them (Kassing & Sanderson, 2009; Lueck, 2015). One market research study found that 63% of adolescents were willing to try a brand suggested by a YouTube influencer, compared to 46% for a brand suggested by a movie or TV celebrity (Arnold, 2017). Even when adolescents recognize user-generated social media posts as a form of marketing, these posts are more effective than brand-generated posts (e.g., Buchanan et al., 2017; Soneji et al., 2018), further suggesting a reduced motivation to resist messages from peers.

Recommendations for an extensive research agenda

The evidence is overwhelming: food marketing is fueling a crisis of poor diet and obesity in children, adolescents, and young adults. Food companies spend billions targeting adolescents and young adults with marketing for calorie-dense HFSS foods, including fast food, SSBs, and snacks, resulting in the highest rates of consuming these same products. Furthermore, food marketers have found new highly appealing ways to reach youth in ways that likely deactivate their skeptical responses to advertising.

Additional research focused on adolescents and young adults is sorely needed to inform effective solutions to this crisis, for several reasons. First, the emphasis on children's understanding of persuasive intent has led to the assumption that adolescent skepticism about marketing means they are less affected. Companies capitalize on this assumption to justify self-regulation of advertising to children only up to age 11 (FTC, 2012), leaving adolescents fair game for advertising of all foods and non-alcoholic beverages. Research demonstrating increased vulnerability of adolescents compared to older adults is essential to support demands for stronger industry self-regulation and government policies to protect children older than age 11 or 12.

Second, research demonstrating that adolescents and adults do not recognize the persuasive intent of "disguised" marketing (e.g., product placements, social media, sponsorships) would provide much-needed evidence to support regulating these practices. Evidence that adolescents are deceived by this marketing (e.g., view it as entertainment or messages from friends) would also support policies to address marketing specifically aimed at youth. Even in the United States, where commercial speech is protected by the First Amendment, government can restrict potentially misleading and deceptive commercial speech (Harris & Graff, 2012). Additional research demonstrating that ad disclosures do not mitigate these effects would enable policymakers to enact more restrictive policy actions.

Finally, research to better understand how food marketing affects adolescents and young adults is essential for identifying effective interventions and policy solutions. Commonly proposed solutions include media literacy (teach youth how marketing works), social marketing campaigns and nutrition education (teach them about healthy eating and why it is important), and healthy food marketing (use marketing to make fruit and vegetables more appealing). However, these solutions do not address the psychological processes that make HFSS marketing so powerful and young people so vulnerable. There is no evidence that increasing skepticism about marketing or understanding the negative health effects of HFSS products would reduce the effects of unhealthy food marketing on adolescents and young adults (Harris, Brownell, et al., 2009).

The FMDM can guide this research agenda (Box 2.2). Numerous research questions remain to assess young people's awareness of food marketing and its persuasive intent; understanding of food marketing effects and how to effectively resist; their cognitive ability to resist short–term rewards in the interest of long–term health; and their motivation to resist, especially when the marketing appeals to their core developmental needs.

BOX 2.2   RESEARCH QUESTIONS TO ASSESS ADOLESCENT AND YOUNG ADULT VULNERABILITIES

Awareness

- Do they consciously attend to or even see non-traditional forms of marketing (e.g., sponsorships, product placements in TV/movies/games)?
- Do they recognize the persuasive intent of these and other non-traditional marketing (e.g., social media posts, influencers)?

Understanding

- Is understanding persuasive intent sufficient to reduce the effects of different forms of marketing, and under what conditions? How do these conditions differ by age and other individual characteristics?
- What are the long-term effects of food marketing exposure on brand and category affective attitudes, and what is the relationship between positive attitudes and consumption?
- Can affective conditioning or other interventions effectively change these attitudes and preferences?
- In what other ways does food marketing affect their health behaviors (e.g., normative beliefs, impulse purchases and consumption, self-identity)?

Ability

- Who has the cognitive ability, and under what circumstances, to resist marketing for products that require forgoing immediate rewards for long-term benefits? How does peer influence affect this ability?
- Are they more susceptible to influence from marketing compared to adults, and does it differ by form of marketing (e.g., image advertising, viral marketing, price/other retail promotions) or product type?

Motivation

- How do different forms of marketing affect their motivation to resist?
- How do other environmental factors (e.g., peers, family) interact with marketing to affect motivations?
- What communications or other interventions effectively increase their motivation to resist (e.g., health promotion campaigns)?

Conclusion

The food industry claims they want to be part of the solution to childhood obesity, while aggressively targeting adolescents and young adults with marketing for products that contribute to obesity and other diet-related diseases. Beliefs that adolescents and young adults are capable of resisting the overwhelmingly unhealthy food environment surrounding them, constrained only by their knowledge and willpower, present a major barrier to improving this environment. Researchers have an important role to play in demonstrating that adolescents remain highly influenced by marketing, which negatively affects their diets and long-term health; that food marketers take advantage of their unique vulnerabilities; and that youth are not equipped to defend against this pervasive negative influence. This research would help increase awareness and concern among parents, policymakers, the public health community – and young people themselves – and create public demand for companies to improve the food marketing environment that places profits over young people's long-term health.

References

Advertising Research Foundation (2008). Innerscope research: A revolution in audience research. Retrieved from http://s3.amazonaws.com/thearf-org-aux-assets/downloads/cnc/engagement/2008-11-19_ARF_Engagement_Innerscope.pdf

Akopyan, M. (2017, April 25). Gatorade is fueling athletic performance, and marketing with innovation. *AList*. Retrieved from https://www.alistdaily.com/strategy/gatorade-fueling-athletic-performance-marketing-innovation/

Albert, D., Chein, J., & Steinberg, L. (2013). The teenage brain: Peer influences on adolescent decision making. *Current Directions in Psychological Science*, *22*, 114–120.

Anderson, M., & Jiang, J. (2018). *Teens, social media & technology 2018*. Retrieved from http://www.pewinternet.org/2018/05/31/teens-social-media-technology-2018

Andreyeva, T., Kelly, I.R., & Harris, J.L. (2011). Exposure to food advertising on television: Associations with children's fast food and soft drink consumption and obesity. *Economics and Human Biology*, *9*, 221–233.

Arain, M., Haque, M., Johal, L., Mathur, P., Nel, W., Rais, A., . . . & Sharma, S. (2013). Maturation of the adolescent brain. *Neuropsychiatric Disease and Treatment*, *9*, 449.

Arnold, A. (2017, June 20). Why YouTube stars influence millennials more than traditional celebrities. *Forbes*. Retrieved from https://www.forbes.com/sites/under30network/2017/06/20/why-youtube-stars-influence-millennials-more-than-traditional-celebrities/#1cd2e1d648c6

Binet, L., & Field, P. (2009). Empirical generalizations about advertising campaign success. *Journal of Advertising Research*, *49*, 130–133.

Bleich, S. N., Vercammen, K. A., Koma, J. W., & Li, Z. (2018). Trends in beverage consumption among children and adults, 2003–2014. *Obesity*, *26*(2), 432–441.

Boush, D.M., Friestad, M., & Rose, G.M. (1994). Adolescent skepticism toward TV advertising and knowledge of advertising tactics. *Journal of Consumer Research*, *21*, 165–175.

Boyland, E. J., Nolan, S., Kelly, B., Tudur-Smith, C., Jones, A., Halford, J. C., & Robinson, E. (2016). Advertising as a cue to consume: A systematic review and meta-analysis of the effects of acute exposure to unhealthy food and nonalcoholic beverage advertising on intake in children and adults. *The American Journal of Clinical Nutrition*, *103*(2), 519–533.

Bragg, M. A., Miller, A. N., Elizee, J., Dighe, S., & Elbel, B. D. (2016). Popular music celebrity endorsements in food and nonalcoholic beverage marketing. *Pediatrics, 138(1)*.

Bragg, M., Miller, A., Roberto, C., Sam, R., Sarda, V., Harris, J. L., & Brownell, K. (2018). Sports sponsorships of food and nonalcoholic beverages. *Pediatrics*, published online.

Bruce, A. S., Bruce, J. M., Black, W. R., Lepping, R. J., Henry, J. M., Cherry, J. B. C., ...Savage, C. R. (2014). Branding and a child's brain: An fMRI study of neural responses to logos. *Social Cognitive and Affective Neuroscience, 9*, 118–122.

Buchanan, L., Kelly, B., & Yeatman, H. (2017). Exposure to digital marketing enhances young adults' interest in energy drinks: An exploratory investigation. *PLOS One, 12*, e0171226.

Buijzen, M., Van Reijmersdal, E. A., & Owen, L. H. (2010). Introducing the PCMC model: An investigative framework for young people's processing of commercialized media content. *Communication Theory, 20(4)*, 427–450.

Burger, K.S., & Stice, E. (2014). Neural responsivity during soft drink intake, anticipation, and advertisement exposure in habitually consuming youth. *Obesity, 22*, 441–450.

Cairns, G., Angus, K., Hastings, G., & Caraher, M. (2013). Systematic reviews of the evidence on the nature, extent and effects of food marketing to children. A retrospective summary. *Appetite, 62*, 209–215.

Chernin, A. (2008). The effects of food advertising on children's preference: Testing the moderating roles of age and gender. *Annals of the Academy of Political Science, 615*, 102–118.

Dietz, W.H. (2017). Obesity and excessive weight gain in young adults: New targets for prevention. *JAMA, 318*, 241–242.

Dotson, M.J., & Hyatt, E.M. (2005). Major influence factors in children's consumer socialization. *Journal of Consumer Marketing, 22*, 35–42.

Dunlop, S., Freeman, B., & Jones, S. C. (2016). Marketing to youth in the digital age: The promotion of unhealthy products and health promoting behaviours on social media. *Media and Communication, 4(3)*, 35–49.

Eisenberg, D., McDowell, J., Berestein, L., Tsiantar, D., & Finan, E. (2002). It's an ad, ad, ad, ad world. *Time, 160*, 38–42.

Elsey, J. & Harris, J.L. (2016). Trends in food and beverage television brand appearances viewed by children and teens from 2009 to 2015. *Public Health Nutrition, 19(11)*, 1928–1933.

Ferraro, R., Bettman, J.R., & Chartrand, T.L. (2008). The power of strangers: The effect of incidental consumer brand encounters on brand choice. *Journal of Consumer Research, 35*, 729–741.

Flegal, K. M., Kruszon-Moran, D., Carroll, M. D., Fryar, C. D., & Ogden, C. L. (2016). Trends in obesity among adults in the United States, 2005 to 2014. *JAMA, 315(21)*, 2284–2291.

Fleming-Milici, F., & Harris, J.L. (2019). Liking, sharing and following: Adolescents' engagement with unhealthy food and beverage brands on social media. Unpublished manuscript.

Freberg, K., Graham, K., McGaughey, K., & Freberg, L. A. (2011). Who are the social media influencers? A study of public perceptions of personality. *Public Relations Review, 37*, 90–92.

Freeman, B., Kelly, B., Baur, L., Chapman, K., Chapman, S., Gill, T., & King, L. (2014). Digital junk: Food and beverage marketing on Facebook. *American Journal of Public Health, 104*, e56–e64.

Friedman, W. (2017, July 18). Traditional TV viewing: Biggest decline from teens, young adults. *MediaPost*. Retrieved from https://www.mediapost.com/publications/article/304495/traditional-tv-viewing-biggest-decline-from-teens.html

Friestad, M., & Wright, P. (1994). The persuasion knowledge model: How people cope with persuasive attempts. *Journal of Consumer Research, 21,* 1–31.

Galvan, A. (2013). The teenage brain: Sensitivity to rewards. *Current Directions in Psychological Science, 22,* 88–93.

Gearhardt, A. N., Yokum, S., Stice, E., Harris, J. L. & Brownell, K. D. (2014). Relation of obesity to neural activation in response to food commercials. *Social Cognitive and Affective Neuroscience, 9*(7), 932–938.

Harris, J. L., Bargh, M. A., & Brownell, K. D. (2009). Priming effects of television food advertising on eating behavior. *Health Psychology, 28,* 404–413.

Harris, J. L., Brownell, K. D., & Bargh, J. A. (2009). The Food Marketing Defense Model: Integrating psychological research to protect youth and inform public policy. *Social Issues and Policy Review, 3,* 211–271.

Harris, J. L., Frazier, W., Fleming-Milici, F., Hubert, P., Rodriguez-Arauz, G., Grier, S., & Appiah. O. (2019). A qualitative assessment of Black and Latino adolescents' attitudes about targeted marketing of unhealthy food and beverages. Unpublished manuscript.

Harris, J. L., Frazier, W., Kumanyika, S., & Ramirez, A.G. (2019). Increasing disparities in food advertising targeted to Hispanic and Black consumers. Retrieved from www.ucon-nruddcenter.org/targetedmarketing

Harris, J. L., Frazier, W., Romo-Palafox, M., Hyary, M., Fleming-Milici, F., Haraghey, K. . . . . & Kalnova, S. (2017). FACTS 2017. Food industry self-regulation after 10 years: Progress and opportunities to improve food advertising to children. Retrieved from http://www.uconnruddcenter.org/files/Pdfs/FACTS-2017_Final.pdf

Harris, J. L. & Graff, S. K. (2012). Ethics of targeting food marketing to young people and the First Amendment: A psychological and legal perspective. *American Journal of Public Health, 102*(2), 214–222.

Harris, J. L., Schwartz, M. B., LoDolce, M., Munsell, C., Fleming-Milici, F., Elsey, J., Liu, S. . . . & Dembek, C. (2014). *Sugary drink FACTS* 2014: Some progress, much room for improvement in marketing to youth. Retrieved from http://sugarydrinkfacts.org/resources/SugaryDrinkFACTS_Report.pdf

Harris, J. L., Schwartz, M. B., Munsell, D. R., Dembek, C., Liu, S., LoDolce, M. . . . . & Kidd, B. (2013). *Fast food FACTS* 2013: Measuring progress in nutrition and marketing to children and teens. Retrieved from http://fastfoodmarketing.org/media/FastFoodFACTS_Report.pdf

Harris, J. L., Schwartz, M. B., Shehan, C., Hyary, M., Appel, J., Haraghey, K., & Li, X. (2015). Snack FACTS 2015: Evaluating snack food nutrition and marketing to youth. Retrieved from http://uconnruddcenter.org/files/Pdfs/SnackFACTS_2015_Fulldraft03.pdf

Hastings, G., Stead, M., McDermott, L., Forsyth, A., MacKintosh, A., Rayner, M.,. . . .Angus, K. (2003). Review of research on the effects of food promotion to children. Retrieved from www.foodstandards.gov.uk/multimedia/pdfs/foodpromotiontochildren1.pdf.

Hawkes, C. (2007). Regulating food marketing to young people worldwide: Trends and policy drivers. *American Journal of Public Health, 97,* 1962–1973.

Healthy Eating Research (2015). Recommendations for responsible food marketing to children. Retrieved from http://healthyeatingresearch.org/wp-content/uploads/2015/01/HER_Food-Marketing-Recomm_1-2015.pdf

Heath, R. (2000). Low involvement processing – a new model of brands and advertising. *International Journal of Advertising, 19,* 287–298.

Institute of Medicine, Committee on Food Marketing and the Diets of Children (2006). *Food Marketing to Children. Threat or Opportunity?* Washington, DC: National Academies Press.

Janiszewski, C. (1993). Preattentive mere exposure effects. *Journal of Consumer Research, 20*, 376–392.

John, D. R. (1999). Consumer socialization of children: A retrospective look at twenty-five years of research. *Journal of Consumer Research, 26*, 183–213.

Kassing, J. W., & Sanderson, J. (2009). 'You're the kind of guy that we all want for a drinking buddy': Expressions of parasocial interaction on FloydLandis.com. *Western Journal of Communication, 73*, 182–203.

Keller, K. L. (2003). Brand synthesis: The multidimensionality of brand knowledge. *Journal of Consumer Research, 29*, 595–600.

Kelly, B., Freeman, B., King, L., Chapman, K., Baur, L. A., & Gill, T. (2016). The normative power of food promotions: Australian children's attachments to unhealthy food brands. *Public health nutrition, 19*(16), 2940–2948.

Kelly, K. J., Slater, M. D., & Karan, D. (2002). Image advertisements' influence on adolescents' perceptions of the desirability of beer and cigarettes. *Journal of Public Policy and Marketing, 21*, 295–304.

Kim, A. J., & Johnson, K. K. (2016). Power of consumers using social media: Examining the influences of brand-related user-generated content on Facebook. *Computers in Human Behavior, 58*, 98–108.

Lueck, J. A. (2015). Friend-zone with benefits: The parasocial advertising of Kim Kardashian. *Journal of Marketing Communications, 21*, 91–109.

Luger, M., Lafontan, M., Bes-Rastrollo, M., Winzer, E., Yumuk, V., & Farpour-Lambert, N. (2017). Sugar-sweetened beverages and weight gain in children and adults: a systematic review from 2013 to 2015 and a comparison with previous studies. *Obesity Facts, 10*(6), 674–693.

McGuire, W. J. (1976). Some internal psychological factors influencing consumer choice. *Journal of Consumer Research, 2*, 302–319.

Mohan, A. M. (2013, April 10). Clarity and boldness mark new Doritos global brand identity. *Packaging World*. Retrieved from https://www.packworld.com/article/food/snacks/chips/clarity-and-boldness-mark-new-doritos-global-brand-identity

Monahan, J. L., Murphy, S. T., & Zajonc, R. B. (2000). Subliminal mere exposure: Specific, general and diffuse effects. *Psychological Science, 11*, 462–466.

Montgomery, K. C., Grier, S. A., Chester, J., & Dorfman, L. (2013). The digital food marketing landscape: challenges for researchers. In *Advances in Communication Research to Reduce Childhood Obesity* (pp. 221–242). New York, NY: Springer.

Moore, E. S. & Lutz, R. L. (2000). Children, advertising and product experiences: A multimethod inquiry. *Journal of Consumer Research, 27*, 31–48.

Nelson, M. C., Story, M., Larson, N. I., Neumark-Sztainer, D., & Lytle, L.A. (2008). Emerging adulthood and college-aged youth: An overlooked age for weight-related behavior change. *Obesity, 16*, 2205–2211.

Nielsen (2017). Millenials on millennials: A look at viewing behavior, distraction and social media stars. Retrieved from https://www.nielsen.com/us/en/insights/news/2017/millennials-on-millennials-a-look-at-viewing-behavior-distraction-social-media-stars.html

Niemeier, H. M., Raynor, H. A., Lloyd-Richardson, E. E., Rogers, M. L., & Wing, R. R. (2006). Fast food consumption and breakfast skipping: predictors of weight gain from adolescence to adulthood in a nationally representative sample. *Journal of Adolescent Health, 39*(6), 842–849.

OFCOM, U.K. (2017). Children and parents: Media use and attitudes report. Retrieved from https://www.ofcom.org.uk/__data/assets/pdf_file/0020/108182/children-parents-media-use-attitudes2017.pdf

Ogden, C. L., Carroll, M. D., Lawman, H. G., Fryar, C. D., Kruszon-Moran, D., Kit, B. K., & Flegal, K. M. (2016). Trends in obesity prevalence among children and adolescents in the United States, 1988–1994 through 2013–2014. *JAMA, 315*(21), 2292–2299.

Paeratakul, S., Ferdinand, D. P., Champagne, C. M., Ryan, D. H., & Bray, G. A. (2003). Fast-food consumption among US adults and children: Dietary and nutrient intake profile. *Journal of the American Dietetic Association, 103*(10), 1332–1338.

Pechmann, C., Levine, L., Loughlin, S., & Leslie, F. (2005). Impulsive and self-conscious: Adolescents' vulnerability to advertising and promotion. *Journal of Public Policy and Marketing, 24,* 202–221.

Petty, R. D., & Andrews, J. C. (2008). Covert marketing unmasked: A legal and regulatory guide for practices that mask marketing messages. *Journal of Public Policy and Marketing, 27,* 7–18.

Powell, L. M., Nguyen, B. T., & Han, E. (2012). Energy intake from restaurants: Demographics and socioeconomics, 2003–2008. *American Journal of Preventive Medicine, 43*(5), 498–504.

Reedy, J., & Krebs-Smith, S. M. (2010). Dietary sources of energy, solid fats, and added sugars among children and adolescents in the United States. *Journal of the American Dietetic Association, 110*(10), 1477–1484.

Rozendaal, E., Lapierre, M., Buijzen, M., & Van Reijmersdal, E. A. (2011). Reconsidering advertising literacy as a defense against advertising effects. *Media Psychology, 14,* 333–354.

Rudd Center. (2013). *Analysis of NPD Group/CREST®/Year and 2 Years Ending* December 2013. Retrieved from https://www.npd.com/wps/portal/npd/us/worldwide/united-states/

Russell, C. A., Norman, A. T., & Heckler, S. E. (2004). The consumption of television programming: Development and validation of the connectedness scale. *Journal of Consumer Research, 31,* 150–161.

Soneji, S., Yang, J., Knutzen, K. E., Moran, M. B., Tan, A. S., ...Choi, K. (2018). Online tobacco marketing and subsequent tobacco use. *Pediatrics,* e20172927.

Statista (2019a). Categories with the largest growth in digital advertising spending in the United States in 2016. Retrieved from https://www.statista.com/statistics/795668/categories-digital-ad-spend-growth-usa/

Statista (2019b). Weekly TV reach in the United States as of March 2018, by age group. Retrieved from https://www.statista.com/statistics/468360/tv-reach-usa/

Steinberg, L., & Monahan, K. C. (2007). Age differences in resistance to peer influence. *Developmental Psychology, 43,* 1531–1543.

Sutherland, L. A., MacKenzie, T., Purvis, L. A., & Dalton, M. (2010). Prevalence of food and beverage brands in movies: 1996–2005. *Pediatrics, 125,* 468–474.

Twenge, J. M., Martin, G. N., & Spitzberg, B. H. (2018). Trends in U.S. adolescents' media use, 1976–2016: The rise of digital media, the decline of TV, and the (near) demise of print. *Psychology of Popular Media Culture,* Advance online publication. dx.doi.org/10.1037/ppm0000203

U.S. Federal Trade Commission (2012). A review of food marketing to children and adolescents: Follow-up report. Retrieved from https://www.ftc.gov/sites/default/files/documents/reports/review-food-marketing-children-and-adolescents-follow-report/121221foodmarketingreport.pdf

Valkenburg, P. M., & Cantor, J. (2001). The development of a child into a consumer. *Applied Developmental Psychology, 26,* 456–468.

Van Reijmersdal, E. A., Boerman, S., Rozendaal, E., & Buijzen, M. (2017). This is advertising! Effects of disclosing television brand placement on adolescents. *Journal of Youth and Adolescence, 46,* 328–342.

Wansink, B. (2003). Using laddering to understand and leverage a brand's equity. *Qualitative Market Research, 6*, 111–118.

Wilson, T. D., & Brekke, N. (1994). Mental contamination and mental correction: Unwanted influences on judgments and evaluations. *Psychological Bulletin, 116*, 117–142.

World Health Organization (2010). Set of recommendations on the marketing of foods and non-alcoholic beverages to children. Retrieved from https://www.who.int/dietphysicalactivity/publications/recsmarketing/en/

World Health Organization (2012). A framework for implementing the set of recommendations on the marketing of foods and non-alcoholic beverages to children. Retrieved from www.who.int/dietphysicalactivity/MarketingFramework2012.pdf

Wright, P. K. (1973). The cognitive processes mediating acceptance of advertising. *Journal of Marketing Research, 10*, 53–62.

Yokum, S., Gearhardt, A. N., Harris, J. L., Brownell, K. D., & Stice, E. (2014). Individual differences in striatum activity to food commercials predict weight gain in adolescents. *Obesity, 22(12)*, 2544–2551.

3

CHILDREN'S RIGHTS WITH REGARD TO FOOD MARKETING

Prof. Dr. Amandine Garde

Introduction

In recent years, there have been increasing calls on states to implement the set of World Health Organization (WHO) recommendations on the marketing of foods and non-alcoholic beverages to children (the Recommendations) with a view to reducing the impact that such marketing has on their health.[1] However, few states to date have done so effectively.[2]

Many factors explain this unfortunate state of affairs, not least the powerful economic interests at stake and the resulting opposition from the food and advertising industries. The slowness with which states have addressed childhood obesity and related non-communicable diseases (NCDs), coupled with the complexity of the response required to change food environments, has led to significant gaps in regulatory frameworks around the world. This slowness contrasts sharply with the reactivity of the food industry to the perceived threat that regulation represents for their economic interests. Shortly after the WHO adopted the Global Strategy on Diet, Physical Activity and Health in 2004,[3] major food business actors adopted a range of voluntary "pledges" and "commitments."[4] However, and notwithstanding the real, perceived, or potential conflicts of interest that self-regulation entails in this policy area, these pledges have not led to a significant reduction in the impact of unhealthy food marketing on children, and research has accumulated on their ineffectiveness.[5]

This chapter argues that states bear the primary responsibility to protect children from harmful marketing: not only do they have an obligation to regulate the commercial practices of the food and advertising industry if these practices are unfair or otherwise harmful, but they also have an obligation to do so effectively to ensure the enjoyment of every child of the highest attainable standard of health.

After discussing the added value of a human rights-based approach to childhood obesity and NCD prevention, this chapter focuses on how states can operationalize human rights to promote the more effective regulation of food marketing to children. It concludes with a few remarks on the implications of a human rights-based approach for industry operators.

This chapter draws in part on some of the core arguments put forward in the report that the Law & NCD Unit at the University of Liverpool was commissioned to write for Unicef, *A Child Rights-Based Approach to Food Marketing: A Guide for Policy Makers*. I would therefore like to acknowledge the contribution of my co-authors, Seamus Byrne, Nikhil Gokani, and Ben Murphy, and invite interested readers to read the full report for a fuller discussion than this chapter allows.[6]

The potential of a rights-based approach to food marketing regulation and NCD prevention

This section highlights the growing number of references to human rights in UN high-profile documents on the prevention and control of NCDs, before focusing more specifically on the role that the UN Convention on the Rights of the Child (CRC) could play in ensuring that states effectively regulate food marketing as part of their childhood obesity prevention strategies.

Food marketing, obesity, NCD prevention, and human rights

From 1998, when the WHO first raised the alarm on rapidly growing rates of childhood obesity,[7] to 2013, when the WHO Global Action Plan for the prevention and control of NCDs for 2013–2020 was adopted,[8] obesity was primarily seen as a public health, and not a human rights, concern. In particular, the 2004 Global Strategy on Diet, Physical Activity and Health did not refer to human rights.[9] The WHO Recommendations did not either.[10] However, since then, we have witnessed a growing momentum, and human rights have featured explicitly – if not necessarily prominently – in most major strategic documents intended to promote healthier diets and prevent diet-related NCDs. The importance of adopting a human rights approach to the prevention and control of NCDs is at the heart of the WHO Global Action Plan which relies on the "human rights approach" as one of its nine overarching principles:

> It should be recognized that the enjoyment of the highest attainable standard of health is one of the fundamental rights of every human being, without distinction of race, colour, sex, language, religion, political or other opinion, national or social origin, property, birth or other status, as enshrined in the Universal Declaration of Human Rights.[11]

Similarly, in its final report, the WHO Commission on Ending Childhood Obesity highlighted that the child's right to health should be the first guiding principle of interventions intended to end childhood obesity:

> Government and society have a moral responsibility to act on behalf of the child to reduce the risk of obesity. Tackling childhood obesity resonates with the universal acceptance of the rights of the child to a healthy life as well as the obligations assumed by State Parties to the Convention of the Rights of the Child.[12]

The international community has since restated its commitment to the prevention of childhood obesity and other NCDs, and the role that the right to health and other related rights could play to this effect.[13]

If the language of human rights has become more prevalent in the global health context, it is noteworthy that human rights organizations have, at the same time, started to refer to the human rights implications of food marketing, obesity, and NCD prevention. In particular, the Committee on the Rights of the Child has noted that the food industry spends billions of dollars on persistent and pervasive marketing strategies promoting unhealthy food to children, and that children's exposure to fast foods should be limited. It has also stated that the marketing of this type of food, *"especially when it is focused on children,"* should be regulated, and the availability in schools and other places controlled.[14] Similarly, references to the need to promote healthy child nutrition and restrict unhealthy food marketing have become more common in the Committee's concluding observations on state parties' reports.[15]

Human rights, child obesity, state obligations, and accountability

A child rights-based approach maintains that the CRC, the most ratified human rights instrument in the world, and other human rights norms should guide all policies that have a foreseeable impact on children, including the regulation of food marketing. It has two defining elements. Firstly, it identifies children as *rights holders* central to any policy discourse and states as the corresponding *duty bearers*, and it works towards strengthening children's capacities to understand and realize their rights and states' capacities to meet their obligations. Secondly, it emphasizes that standards and principles derived from international human rights treaties, and the CRC more specifically, should guide all policies that have the potential to impact upon children.

As such, *a children's rights approach guarantees a degree of accountability by imposing legal obligations on states*, making effective remedies more likely where rights are violated. Support for monitoring the commitments made by states is an intrinsic part of follow-up to ratification of the CRC, including through public and independent assessments of performance, with the help of recommendations from the Committee on the Rights of the Child. A children's rights approach therefore has the potential to translate the commitments and obligations established in the CRC into operable, durable, and realizable entitlements. Moreover, the weight that rights discourses entail adds to the utility of a rights-based approach. As children's rights are inalienable and universal, there is an inherent legitimacy to the language of human rights. Thus, children's rights arguments can ensure that an issue is given special consideration in public policy, and competing interests can be granted lesser relative weight if they are incompatible with children's rights.[16]

More specific, the *Bauducco* case from Brazil illustrates the potential that a child rights-based approach offers to limit the exposure of children to unhealthy food marketing. In 2007, Alana initiated a legal challenge against Bauducco's "*It's Shrek Time*" advertising campaign.[17] In this campaign, children were encouraged to collect four different wristwatches with the picture of Shrek and other licensed cartoon characters from the movie. Children could obtain each of these watches by exchanging five labels found on packs of cakes and cookies, together with a small additional amount of money. In its decision of 10 March 2016, the São Paulo Court of Justice held that the marketing campaign was illegal and deceptive, as it took advantage of the naivety of children by advertising unhealthy food directly to them. It therefore rejected Bauducco's claim that the promotion was directed at parents rather than children. It also noted that children were especially vulnerable, and that Article 227 of the Brazilian Constitution enshrined, as an absolute priority, state protection of children, safeguarding them from any form of exploitation.[18] Even though the Constitution also grants freedom of expression to advertisers, this right can be restricted in law, particularly marketing strategies should be illegal if they exploit the poor discernment of children and condition the purchase of a thematic watch to the acquisition of a given quantity of food products. Bauducco's appeal to the Superior Court was dismissed and the conviction upheld. This decision sets the precedent that food advertising directed at children, either directly or indirectly, can be abusive.

> The position of the court is in line with the UN Declaration on the Rights of the Child and with international recommendations that are gaining more prominence on account of the rising consmption of ultra-processed foods – linked to the occurrence of obesity-related diseases.[19]

Overall, however, little guidance had been provided to states on how they could operationalize the rights enshrined in the CRC and regulate the marketing of food to protect children from its harmful influence. Alongside a growing body of academic research focusing on unhealthy food marketing as an important children's rights issue,[20] Unicef and the WHO have started to fill in the gap.[21] Whilst Unicef has become more interested in the prevention of child obesity, the WHO seems to have embraced more systematically the potential human rights can offer to better prevent and control obesity and NCDs.[22] The coordinated action of various UN agencies is most welcome to draw on their complementary expertise and harness this potential.

Operationalizing human rights to protect children from unhealthy food marketing

After establishing the importance of adopting a dynamic interpretation of the CRC, this section argues that the Recommendations should inform how states should regulate food marketing as part of their mandate to respect, protect, and fulfill children's rights, particularly their right to the enjoyment of the highest attainable standard of health (often referred to as the right to health).[23]

For a dynamic interpretation of the CRC

The right to health is a universal human right.[24] In particular, Article 24 of the CRC requires that "*States Parties recognize the right of the child to the enjoyment of the highest attainable standard of health and to facilities for the treatment of illness and rehabilitation of health*" and, more specifically, that they "*take appropriate measures to diminish infant and child mortality [and] to combat disease and malnutrition, through, inter alia, the provision of adequate nutritious foods.*" This provision must be interpreted broadly in light of the General Comment on Article 24 of the Committee on the Rights of the Child, which is entrusted with the interpretation and monitoring of the CRC, as:

> an inclusive right, extending not only to timely and appropriate prevention, health promotion, curative, rehabilitative and palliative services, but also to a right to grow and develop to their full potential and live in conditions that enable them to attain the highest standard of health through the implementation of programmes that address the underlying determinants of health.[25]

States must fulfill the child's right to health to the maximum extent of their available resources and, where needed, within the framework of international cooperation.[26] The notion of the "highest attainable standard of health" takes into account both the child's biological, social, cultural, and economic conditions and the resources available to the state, supplemented by resources made available by other sources, including non-governmental organizations and the international community. Even though the right to health is not a right to be healthy as such, it nonetheless amounts to a right to the conditions and services that ensure the enjoyment of the best health standards attainable under existing circumstances. Consequently, it mandates states to provide the opportunity for every child to enjoy the highest attainable standard of health, as opposed to any standard of health.

Neither Article 24 CRC nor any other provisions of the CRC refer explicitly to "obesity." This should not come as a surprise, bearing in mind that the CRC was adopted in 1989, a few years before childhood obesity came to be seen as a major global public health problem. Broadly defined, the right to health has an important role to play in the prevention of diseases, including NCDs, which can only be effectively prevented if the environments in which children live are durably changed to promote healthier choices.[27] The wording of Article 24 CRC supports such a wide interpretation of the right to health and its relevance to NCD and obesity prevention.[28] In particular, Article 24(2) CRC refers to the duty of states to take appropriate measures to reduce infant and child mortality, and to combat disease and malnutrition through the provision of adequate nutritious foods, among other actions. In light of the clear emerging international consensus that states should address both undernutrition and overnutrition,[29] there are compelling reasons why the CRC and other relevant human rights norms on the right to health, on the right to food, and on other related rights should be interpreted to ensure that states are accountable for their failure to develop effective obesity prevention strategies, of which it is now well established that unhealthy food marketing restrictions are an effective component. As noted by the Committee on the Rights of the Child, *"children's health is affected by a variety of factors, many of which have changed during the past 20 years and are likely to continue to evolve in the future."*[30] States are therefore encouraged to prioritize issues that have received little attention to date and should ensure, among other things, the availability of safe and nutritionally adequate food and a healthy and safe environment. A dynamic interpretation of the CRC is therefore warranted, and states should address health concerns affecting children at a given point in time, and not at the time the Convention was adopted, when obesity was not seen as a major global public health issue.

For a comprehensive implementation of the Recommendations

The central argument that the Unicef report has advanced is that the Recommendations should guide the interpretation of what the CRC and international human rights treaties require from states parties to ensure that they uphold their legal obligation to respect, protect, and fulfill children's rights from harmful business practices. Even though the Recommendations are not legally binding, they reflect on existing evidence and call on states to ensure that children are protected from harmful marketing. To this extent, they should be granted much more weight in the interpretation of human rights provisions than has been done to date. It is necessary to reconcile public health and human rights discourses as mutually reinforcing.[31]

The duty of member states to uphold the right of children to the highest standard of attainable health, the right to adequate food, and several other related rights requires the full implementation of the WHO Recommendations. In turn, this requires that the scope of relevant food marketing restrictions is clearly defined. Firstly, states should adopt an independent evidence-based nutrient profiling system to determine which food is unhealthy (and should not be marketed) and which food is healthy (and may be marketed). Secondly, they should define the key notion of "marketing to children" broadly to include both direct and indirect marketing. The evaluation of existing regulatory frameworks which limit the exposure of children to advertising in and around children's programs has shown that such a narrow focus allows for significant investment shifts from food and advertising business actors from regulated to unregulated programs, leaving them exposed to high levels of unhealthy food marketing. As the Recommendations clearly emphasize, the more comprehensive the restrictions on unhealthy food marketing, the more effective they are likely to be in protecting children from its harmful effects.[32] Therefore, beyond the regulation of television advertising, it is important to ensure that all settings where children gather are free from all forms of unhealthy food marketing; this specifically requires that they regulate sponsorship by the food industry of sports and cultural events attended by a high number of children. Similarly, the growing use of digital media requires that children are protected from exposure online too.

Finally, a children's rights approach also embraces international cooperation to ensure that the effectiveness of national measures intended to protect children from unhealthy food marketing is not limited as a result of cross-border marketing which states will find difficult to regulate unilaterally. The problem is all the more acute in regions that have close cultural and linguistic ties, and is likely to become even more so with the rapid development of digital marketing.[33]

All in all, a children's rights approach requires that the measures adopted by member states be goal-oriented, i.e., they must effectively restrict the exposure of children to unhealthy food marketing and the power such marketing has over them: the more comprehensive the implementation of the Recommendations, the more in line states will be with their obligations under the CRC.[34] This will, in turn, help to provide a healthier environment and support parents in the performance of their child-rearing responsibilities.[35]

Ultimately, a human rights-based approach may help galvanize the political will required to implement the Recommendations comprehensively in line with what a human rights-based approach requires. In particular, a child rights-based approach to food marketing regulation requires that the outstanding challenges and loopholes identified are both recognized and effectively addressed at national and/or regional levels. For this, the key notions underpinning the implementation of the Recommendations should be defined broadly and independently of vested interests to ensure the effective protection of children from the harmful impact that unhealthy food marketing has on them; and that the risk of investment shift should be considerably limited. Indeed, only comprehensive approaches can ensure that marketing does not "migrate":

- from regulated to unregulated programs (e.g., from children's programs to programs with a high children's audience in absolute numbers);
- from regulated to unregulated media (e.g., from broadcast media to digital media, packaging, or sponsorship);
- from regulated to unregulated marketing techniques (e.g., from licensed to equity brand characters); and
- from regulated to unregulated settings (e.g., from schools to other settings where children gather).

Furthermore, a children's rights approach reinforces the need for states to protect all children, including adolescents. While the CRC may recognize that children's vulnerabilities vary from one stage of childhood to another, it applies to all children – a child being defined as every human being under 18 years old – and does not exempt states from their obligations to protect them from harm, including the harm that unhealthy food marketing causes.[36]

States need to anticipate the objections to food marketing regulation they are bound to encounter at the various stages of the policy process, from adoption to implementation, monitoring, and evaluation. Several of these objections will be grounded in international trade law (broadly construed to include international investment law). The rights implicated in the childhood obesity and NCD prevention debate are not absolute and must take account of competing rights and interests; similarly, the rights and interests invoked against food marketing regulation are not absolute either. An assessment of competing rights and interests should therefore be undertaken to determine where the balance should lie. This is discussed further in the next section.[37] However, and in conformity with their obligation under Article 3(1) of the CRC, states must take "*the best interests of the child*" as "*a primary consideration*" and ensure that children's rights are placed at the center of the policy process leading up to the implemention of the Recommendations. This will require the adoption of robust food marketing restrictions which, in itself, presupposes that states have managed to build a consensus of relevant stakeholders both within and beyond government.[38]

Human rights and corporate social responsibility: what role for industry?

Since the adoption of the 2004 WHO Global Strategy on Diet, Physical Activity and Health, the food industry has been keen to be perceived as a "partner" in the global fight against obesity. However, it is clear that their attitude has been rather ambivalent and their partnership extremely erratic, as the challenges they have mounted against food marketing restrictions threatening their high profit margins demonstrate.

Food marketing and industry pledges to promote food "responsibly" to children

The review of internal corporate social responsibility documents suggests that food business actors do not yet consider the impact of unhealthy food marketing on children as a human rights issue and they do not consider it necessary to assess the impact of their commercial practices on children in their corporate social responsibility reports.[39] Nevertheless, they have recognized that they should be responsible business actors and play their part in the prevention of childhood obesity.

> United Nations and World Health Organization strategies on global public health recognize that efforts to help people improve their diets and health require a whole-of-society effort and actions by all stakeholders – including the private sector. We take this responsibility seriously and have committed to do our part and to work in collaboration with all stakeholders in the execution of our commitments and the realization of the global public health strategies of the UN and WHO.[40]

To this effect, several major multinational food companies have adopted joint pledges or commitments, in particular to promote food "responsibly" to children. However, these pledges have been largely ineffective in restricting the exposure of children to unhealthy food marketing and the overall impact that such marketing has had on their health and their rights. If there is a high level of compliance with them, the thresholds they adopt to define their scope make them extremely ill suited as instruments of child rights protection. If food business actors have increased the level of their commitment under public pressure, they have never done so to the level the Recommendations would require, leaving major loopholes and, accordingly, major opportunities for investment shift from self-regulated programs / media / marketing techniques / settings to those not covered by the EU Pledge. For example, the age of the child to be protected remains below 12; the audience threshold to determine whether a program is "to children" remains high, at 35% (though down to 50% originally); and several media or marketing techniques used to promote unhealthy food to children are not covered, including product packaging, product displays at points of sale, sponsorship. . . In particular, the food industry refuses to accept that they should avoid using equity brand characters on the promotion of unhealthy food, even though these characters have, by definition, been designed for marketing purposes to influence children's preferences and purchase requests.

It must be acknowledged that the international community has not been sufficiently clear in where the red lines should lie. Significant ambiguity remains regarding the extent to which food business actors can promote food "responsibly" to children,[41] and this ambiguity does not sit well with the imperative of adopting a human rights approach to obesity and NCD prevention.

The major real, perceived, or potential conflicts of interests which character-
ize this policy area strongly suggest that self-regulation is not well suited at all
for the effective regulation of food marketing and the protection of children's
rights. As Anand Grover, then United Nations Special Rapporteur on the
right to health, vividly stated in 2014:

> Owing to the inherent problems associated with self-regulation and public–
> private partnerships, there is a need for States to adopt laws that prevent
> companies from using insidious marketing strategies. The responsibility to
> protect the enjoyment of the right to health warrants State intervention in
> situations when third parties, such as food companies, use their position
> to influence dietary habits by directly or indirectly encouraging unhealthy
> diets, which negatively affect people's health. Therefore, States have a
> positive duty to regulate unhealthy food advertising and the promotion
> strategies of food companies. Under the right to health, States are especially
> required to protect vulnerable groups such as children from violations of
> their right to health.[42]

Ultimately, if self-regulation has failed to significantly reduce the overall
exposure of children to unhealthy food marketing, a child rights-based approach
mandates that states recognize its inherent limits and that they use their regulatory powers to ensure that the Recommendations are effectively implemented and
child health and children's rights protected from harmful commercial practices.

Challenging evidence-based food marketing restrictions

The good faith on which "partnerships" with food business actors rest is
questionable, and suspicion increases as one becomes aware of the vigorous
opposition that these actors are prepared to mount against any robust, evidence-
based restrictions on unhealthy food marketing. Major food companies, often
with the support of the advertising industry, have attempted to avoid regulation in the first instance by minimizing the contribution that food marketing
makes to unhealthy diets and therefore childhood obesity, whilst exaggerating
the contribution that marketing plays in promoting consumer choice, liberal
market economies and prosperity, often invoking the specter of overly paternal-
ist state regulatory interventions in personal choices and consumer autonomy.
Furthermore, once regulation has been adopted in areas where the Pledges do
not apply, food business actors have relentlessly challenged such measures to try
and restrict their scope and, in turn, their effectiveness.[43]

Thinking by analogy is useful, drawing on the experience derived from the
analysis of the opposition that tobacco and alcohol control strategies have encoun-
tered, in order to anticipate the challenges that states are likely to face as they
increasingly regulate the marketing of unhealthy food to children. States do so

more comprehensively and they therefore comply more effectively with their human rights obligations. Tobacco and alcohol manufacturers have relied on a broad range of legal arguments, ranging from fundamental rights (e.g., advertising is often protected as a form of commercial expression) to trade arguments (e.g., advertising measures would constitute unnecessary restrictions to European Union, World Trade Organization, or other form of international trade law). And they have invoked these many legal arguments before every possible forum, from national courts or regional courts (e.g., the Court of Justice of the European Union) to global dispute settlement bodies (e.g., the World Trade Organization Dispute Settlement Body, or international arbitration tribunals). One should therefore expect that the more states are going to restrict the possibilities for food business actors to promote unhealthy food as they wish, the more their regulatory frameworks are going to be challenged. The public health community should therefore stand ready for these challenges.

It is important to emphasize that neither the rights of industry operators to free commercial expression and intellectual property nor their claims that regulation would create obstacles to trade are absolute. They can be, and are routinely, restricted on grounds of public health, consumer and child protection. Importantly, under European and international trade law, member states have a broad margin of discretion to restrict commercial rights (to free commercial expression or intellectual property) to protect the health of their citizens, not least children who are particularly vulnerable to commercial practices. They must, however, ensure that the measures they adopt to implement the Recommendations are non-discriminatory and necessary to achieve the intended objective they pursue.

There is a vast amount of case law on the relationship between free trade and public health protection. This is why the public health community, assisted by competent lawyers, must thoroughly engage with existing trade rules as interpreted by relevant courts, tribunals, and dispute settlement bodies. This requires that public health experts work closely with trade experts to ensure that they understand these rules and their rationale and can develop an effective strategy from the moment they start to envisage the design of regulatory measures such as unhealthy food marketing restrictions. The more member states understand the constraints deriving from international trade law, the more they can maximize the opportunities that the law offers to effectively prevent NCDs, and childhood obesity more specifically. A human rights approach to childhood obesity and NCD prevention calls for an enquiry into how the right to the highest attainable standard of health and other human rights can be used to counter the arguments put forward by business actors. The tide is turning. While human rights may have traditionally been relied upon by business actors to protect their interests from unwanted health-promoting measures, they are now – and should increasingly be – invoked by public health policymakers to develop and defend effective, evidence-based NCD prevention strategies with the imperative of ensuring a high level of public health protection in all policies.[44]

The responsibility of food business actors to respect children's rights

Finally, business actors themselves have a responsibility under the United Nations Guiding Principles on Business and Human Rights to ensure they do not violate human rights.[45] The food industry should therefore ensure that their marketing practices respect the rights enshrined in the CRC and refrain from marketing unhealthy food to children, including adolescents. Such responsibility therefore goes beyond the pledges that food business actors have adopted to date: a more comprehensive approach is warranted.

Where business actors fail to fulfill this responsibility, states must take all necessary measures to facilitate the enjoyment of human rights. This includes the positive duty to regulate unhealthy food marketing, as incumbent in the obligation to protect and fulfill the child's right to the highest attainable standard of health and other related rights.[46]

Conclusion

As the most ratified human rights instrument in the world, the CRC provides the basis for a normative children's rights approach to obesity and NCD prevention, by establishing the obligations of state and the responsibilities of other stakeholders, particularly business actors. As the Recommendations are based on independent, consistent, and unequivocal evidence that children's health is negatively influenced by unhealthy food marketing, they should inform the interpretation of the CRC and other human instruments. States should adopt comprehensive restrictions to the marketing of unhealthy food to promote healthier diets and therefore contribute to more effective childhood obesity prevention strategies. It is only then that they will have fully upheld their human rights obligations.

The potential of rights-based arguments remains largely untapped – though there are signs that the connection between the human rights and the public health communities is intensifying. A human rights-based approach provides an opportunity to build strategic alliances, coalitions, and networks with other actors who share a similar vision and pursue common objectives. In relation to childhood obesity, a children's rights approach is likely to foster the involvement of a broad range of actors who may not have viewed the issue of marketing of unhealthy food to children as raising children's rights concerns. In turn, this is likely to help galvanize political will and increase pressure on states to ensure that they do comply with their human rights obligations, not least their obligations under the CRC.

Notes

1 WHO, *A set of recommendations on the marketing of foods and non-alcoholic beverages to children*, WHO (Geneva, 2010).
2 For an overview of the implementation worldwide of the Recommendations, see Kraak, Vivica, et al., Progress achieved in restricting the marketing of high-fat, sugary and salty

food and beverage products to children, *Bulletin of the World Health Organization* 2016; *94* (7): 540–548. For a review of their implementation in the European region, see WHO, *Evaluating implementation of the WHO set of recommendations on the marketing of foods and non-alcoholic beverages to children. Progress, challenges and guidance for next steps in the WHO European Region* (WHO, Copenhagen, 2018); and in the East Mediterranean region, see WHO, *Implementing the WHO recommendations on the marketing of food and non-alcoholic beverages to children in the Eastern Mediterranean region* (WHO, Cairo, 2018).

3 WHO, *Global strategy on diet, physical activity and health* (Geneva, 2004). On the development of this strategy, see Kaare Norum, World Health Organization's global strategy on diet, physical activity and health: the process behind the scenes, *Scandinavian Journal of Nutrition* 2005; *49*: 83.

4 See in particular the International Food Alliance Beverage (IFBA) Pledge and all related regional pledges: https://ifballiance.org/. "*We innovate, empower and collaborate to help consumers eat balanced diets and live healthier lives.*"

5 For example, see Galbraith-Emami Sarah, Lobstein Tim, The impact of initiatives to limit the advertising of food and beverage products to children: a systematic review, *Obesity Review* 2013; December 14(12): 960–974.

6 Unicef, *A child rights-based approach to food marketing: a guide for policy makers* (Unicef, Geneva, 2018).

7 See the WHO Consultation on Obesity carried out in 1999 and published in *Obesity: preventing and managing the global epidemic* (WHO, Geneva, first published in 2000 and reprinted in 2004), Technical Report Series 894.

8 WHO, *Global action plan for the prevention and control of noncommunicable diseases, 2013– 2020* (WHO, Geneva, 2013).

9 In this respect, the Global Strategy differs from the Framework Convention on Tobacco Control (WHO, Geneva, 2003), which does refer to the right to health.

10 The WHO *Framework for implementing the recommendations* (WHO, Geneva, 2012), which put some flesh on the bones of the Recommendations, refers in passing to the CRC without, however, framing the issue of obesity as a child rights concern.

11 WHO Global Action Plan, at p. 12.

12 WHO, *Report of the commission on ending childhood obesity* (WHO, Geneva, 2016), pp. 8, 10, 40. To provide guidance to the Commission, two ad hoc working groups were convened: on the science and evidence for ending childhood obesity; and on implementation, monitoring and accountability frameworks.

13 In particular, the Political Declaration that concluded the Third UN High Level Meeting on Non-Communicable Diseases on 27 September 2018 explicitly reaffirmed the right to health (at paragraph 3) and the primary role and responsibility of governments at all levels in responding to the challenge of NCDs by developing adequate national multi-sectoral responses for their prevention and control, and promoting and protecting the right of everyone to the enjoyment of the highest attainable standard of physical and mental health (at paragraph 15): United Nations, Resolution adopted by the General Assembly, 10 October 2018, A/RES/73/2.

14 Committee on the Rights of the Child, *General comment no. 15 on the right of the child to the enjoyment of the highest attainable standard of health*, CRC/C/GC/15, United Nations, 17 April 2013, para. 47.

15 Unicef, *A child rights-based approach to food marketing: a guide for policy makers* contains a more systematic review of the references to childhood obesity and food marketing in UN documents. So does Katharina Ó Cathaoir's PhD thesis: *A children's rights approach to obesogenic marketing* (University of Copenhagen, 2017).

16 Unicef, *A child rights-based approach to food marketing: a guide for policy makers*, section 3.2.

17 Alana is a non-profit civil society organization whose mission is to "*honour children*" and works on projects which pursue the essential conditions for a happy, fulfilling childhood. This legal challenge as part of its *Crianca e Consumo* (Children and Consumerism) project, which strives to minimize and prevent the harm that may be inflicted by children-direct advertisement (www.criancaeconsumo.org.br).

18 The Brazilian Constitution also establishes consumer protection as a fundamental right, which requires that the state should defend consumer interests.

19 http://criancaeconsumo.org.br/acoes/pandurata-alimentos-bauducco-promocao-gulosos-shrek/.

20 For example, see Tobin, John, Beyond the supermarket shelf: using a rights-based approach to address children's health needs, *International Journal of Children's Rights* 2006; *14* (3): 275–306; Garde, Amandine, Advertising regulation and the protection of children-consumers in the European Union: in the best interest of . . . commercial operators?, *International Journal of Children's Rights* 2011; *19* (3): 523–45; Handsley, Elizabeth et al., A children's rights perspective on food advertising to children, *International Journal of Children's Rights* 2014; *22* (1): 93–134; Mills, Lize, *Considering the best interests of the child when marketing food to children: an analysis of the South African regulatory framework* (PhD thesis, Stellenbosch University, 2016); Ó Cathaoir, Katharina, *A children's rights approach to obesogenic marketing* (PhD thesis, University of Copenhagen, 2017).

21 Up to 2015, Unicef had been remarkably silent on childhood obesity, in sharp contrast with its involvement in the development of the Code of Marketing of Breastmilk Substitutes in the late 1970s / early 1980s. One could speculate on what initiated a change of attitude – perhaps the establishment of the UN Interagency Task Force on NCDs. The Task Force held a session on NCDs and the law (Sixth Meeting, February 2016), and one NCDs and human rights (Eighth Meeting, February 2017), leading to the establishment of the NCDs and the law program.

22 See, in particular: WHO Regional Office for Europe, *Tackling food marketing to children in a digital world: trans-disciplinary perspectives* (WHO, Copenhagen, 2016); WHO Regional Office for the East Mediterranean, *Implementing the WHO recommendations on the marketing of food and non-alcoholic beverages to children in the Eastern Mediterranean region* (WHO, Cairo, 2018); and WHO Regional Office for Europe, *Evaluating implementation of the WHO set of recommendations on the marketing of foods and non-alcoholic beverages to children. Progress, challenges and guidance for next steps in the WHO European region* (WHO, Copenhagen, 2018).

23 Importantly, beyond its negative impact on the right to health, the marketing of unhealthy food consumed by children also has a negative impact on other rights, including the rights to food, survival and development, education, information, rest, leisure, recreation and cultural activities, privacy, and non-discrimination. For a fuller discussion of the variety of rights negatively affected by unhealthy food marketing, see Unicef, *A child rights-based approach to food marketing: a guide for policy makers*, specifically section 3.3 and the Annex; and Ó Cathaoir, Katharina, *A children's rights approach to obesogenic marketing* (PhD thesis, University of Copenhagen; 2017).

24 On the right to health, see in particular: Toebes, Brigit, *The right to health as a human right in international law* (Intersentia, 1999), and Tobin, John, *The right to health in international law* (Oxford University Press, 2012).

25 Committee on the Rights of the Child, General Comment No. 15 (2013) on the right of the child to the enjoyment of the highest attainable standard of health (Article 24), CRC/C/GC/15 (at paragraph 1). The Committee on Economic, Social and Cultural Rights has done the same in relation to Article 12 of the International Covenant on Economic, Social and Cultural Rights: General Comment No. 14 (2000) on the right of everyone to the enjoyment of the highest attainable standard of physical and mental health (Article 12), E/C.12/2000/4.

26 Article 4 CRC.

27 This was forcefully reiterated by the WHO Commission on Ending Childhood Obesity (ECHO) in: WHO, *Report of the Commission on Ending Childhood Obesity* (WHO, January 2016).

28 As Tobin notes, this stems clearly not only from the text of Article 24 itself, but also from the drafting history of the CRC: Tobin, John, *The right to health in international law* (Oxford University Press, 2012), p. 131.

29 See, in particular, UN General Assembly, *Transforming our world: the 2030 agenda for sustainable development*, A/RES/70/1, New York, 25 September 2015; UN General Assembly, '*United Nations decade of action on nutrition (2016–2025)*', A/RES/70/259, 15 April 2016; and more recently Swinburn, Boyd, et al., The global syndemic of obesity, undernutrition, and climate change: *The Lancet* commission report, *The Lancet* 2019; *39* (10173): 791–846.

30 Committee on the Rights of the Child, *General comment no. 15 on the right of the child to the enjoyment of the highest attainable standard of health*, CRC/C/GC/15, United Nations, 17 April 2013, para. 5.

31 Chapter in Burci, Gian Luca, and Toebes, Brigit (eds), *Research handbook on global health law* (Edward Elgar, 2018)..

32 The need for comprehensive marketing restrictions, tackling both exposure and power, is discussed extensively both in Unicef, *A child rights-based approach to food marketing: a guide for policy makers*, and in WHO Regional Office for Europe, *Evaluating implementation of the WHO set of recommendations on the marketing of foods and non-alcoholic beverages to children. Progress, challenges and guidance for next steps in the WHO European region* (WHO, Copenhagen, 2018).

33 WHO Regional Office for the East Mediterranean, *Implementing the WHO recommendations on the marketing of food and non-alcoholic beverages to children in the Eastern Mediterranean region* (WHO, Cairo, 2018), section 3.3.

34 Unicef, *A child rights-based approach to food marketing: a guide for policy makers*.

35 Under Article 5 CRC, states are expected to support parents' role, respecting "*the responsibilities, rights and duties of parents . . . to provide, in a manner consistent with the evolving capacities of the child, appropriate direction and guidance*" in exercising their rights. In relation to food marketing more specifically, see section 3.3 of the Unicef report; and Ó Cathaoir, Katharina, *A children's rights approach to obesogenic marketing*, which discusses this point more extensively and refers to the work of Kent George, Children's right to adequate nutrition, *International Journal of Children's Rights* 1993; *1* (2): 133–154.

36 On this point, see also Unicef, *A child rights-based approach to food marketing: a guide for policy makers*, and WHO Regional Office for Europe, *Evaluating implementation of the WHO set of recommendations on the marketing of foods and non-alcoholic beverages to children. Progress, challenges and guidance for next steps in the WHO European region* (WHO, Copenhagen, 2018).

37 For a more extensive discussion, see Garde, Amandine, Law and non-communicable diseases prevention: maximizing opportunities by understanding constraints, in Burci, Gian Luca, and Toebes, Brigit (eds), *Research handbook on global health law* (Edward Elgar, 2018).

38 The implications of the principle of the best interest of the child for states when implementing the WHO Recommendations are discussed more fully in the Unicef report, section 4.1.

39 Ó Cathaoir, Katharina, Children's right to freedom from obesity: responsibilities of the food industry, *Nordic Journal of Human Rights* 2018; *36* (2): 109–131.

40 https://ifballiance.org/commitments/collaboration.

41 Garde, Amandine, et al., Implementing the WHO recommendations whilst avoiding real, perceived or potential conflicts of interest, *European Journal of Risk Regulation* 2017; *8* (2): 237.

42 Grover, Anand, *Unhealthy foods, non-communicable diseases and the right to health*, A/HRC/26/31, Report of the Special Rapporteur on the right of everyone to the enjoyment of the highest attainable standard of physical and mental health, United Nations, 1 April 2014, para. 25.

43 The resistance to the Chilean ban on the use of equity brand characters and other marketing techniques of particular appeal to children for the promotion of unhealthy food is a striking example.

44 Garde, Amandine, Law and non-communicable diseases prevention: maximizing opportunities by understanding constraints, in Burci, Gian Luca, and Toebes, Brigit (eds), *Research handbook on global health law* (Edward Elgar, 2018).
45 Ruggie, John, *Guiding principles on business and human rights: implementing the United Nations "Protect, Respect and Remedy" framework*, Report of the Special Representative of the Secretary-General on the issue of human rights and transnational corporations and other business enterprises, A/HRC/17/31, United Nations, 21 March 2011. On the relationship between food marketing and the Guiding Principles, see Løvhaug, Anna Lene, *Exploring food marketing to children in the context of the UN Guiding Principles Reporting Framework: a salient human rights issue?* (Master's thesis, Oslo, 2017).
46 Unicef report, section 4.2.

4

REGULATIONS AND THEIR EFFECTIVENESS

Dr. Bridget Kelly

Children's exposure to persuasive promotions for unhealthy foods and beverages is established as a causal factor that contributes to children's poor diets and childhood overweight and obesity [1]. There is growing evidence globally on the necessary actions to address this issue, including regulatory provisions to restrict children's exposure to unhealthy food marketing and the persuasive content of this marketing. Such evidence highlights the primacy of government-led, comprehensive marketing restrictions [2]. In this context, 'comprehensive' refers to the application of marketing restrictions across all media and settings. However, little effective action has been taken globally that is aligned with evidence of best-practice actions; most actions have been industry-led and narrowly focused on restrictions to specific media or marketing techniques.

This chapter aims to describe options and best practices for regulatory interventions to protect children from unhealthy food marketing, their apparent relative effectiveness and the state of regulatory action globally to date. First, we briefly reiterate the problem of food marketing to children, which was the focus of the first part of this book. Second, we present policy options or solutions for protecting children from the harmful impacts of food marketing, including intra-personal and socio-environmental solutions. Third, focusing on regulatory options, the chapter describes the relative effectiveness or potential effectiveness of food marketing regulation, including government- and private sector-led arrangements. Finally, the role of civil society and academia in progressing an effective regulatory agenda will be discussed.

The problem

Children's exposure to unhealthy food marketing is now widely accepted by leading international health organisations to be a causal factor contributing to childhood overweight and obesity. As established in the earlier chapters of this book, pervasive exposure to persuasive food marketing influences children's food knowledge, preferences and behaviours. Given that the most frequently promoted products are the antithesis of dietary recommendations, comprising predominantly ultra-processed foods and beverages high in added fat, sugar and/ or sodium (referred to here as 'unhealthy'), this link between food marketing exposure and food-related attitudes and behaviours poses a threat to children's diets and healthy nutrition globally. Evidence on the impact of unhealthy food marketing on childhood obesity is considered by leading global health authorities to be unequivocal [1].

Marketing is broadly defined and includes advertising, sponsorship and promotions, each encompassing a range of media platforms or settings [3]. Contemporary marketing campaigns typically apply an integrated communications approach, using a range of marketing platforms and techniques in parallel to achieve maximum impact [4]. For example, campaigns may include a mass broadcast media advertisement to achieve widespread brand awareness, product promotions to drive short-term sales and targeted online behavioural marketing to build long-term brand attachment and loyalty.

Together, the combination of media platforms or settings and the techniques used within marketing communications determine the effectiveness of marketing campaigns. Campaign effectiveness is a consequence of: (1) exposure to the message; and (2) the persuasive power of the message [5]. Exposure refers to the reach and frequency of contact with marketing messages, and is a function of the media platforms used, marketing expenditure and children's media use behaviours. Persuasive power of marketing relates to the actual content and design of marketing messages. Frequent exposure to persuasive messages is the endgame of marketing campaigns.

An appreciation of the array of marketing media and techniques, and their integration, is important in building solutions to protect children from unhealthy food marketing. The very nature of contemporary integrated marketing communications means that the restriction of marketing a limited set of media or techniques would simply result in a migration in marketing budgets and efforts to other less regulated media (e.g. from television to digital media) or techniques (e.g. from licensed characters to brand equity characters). As such, comprehensive restrictions that cover all forms of marketing are promulgated.

The solution

There are two major approaches for protecting children from food marketing, representing an upstream and a mid-stream approach. First, upstream policies aim to shape the economic, social and physical environments, including the food environment. Second, mid-stream policies directly act on behaviours, across populations [6].

In relation to food marketing, the *socio-environmental (upstream) approach* seeks to reduce children's exposure to, and the power of, unhealthy food marketing by altering the media environment. Alternatively, the intention of *behavioural (mid-stream) approaches* is to reduce the impact that marketing has on individuals, by focusing on inter-personal solutions. This includes, for example, increasing marketing literacy to build awareness and understanding of the harms and manipulation caused by unhealthy food marketing, with the aim of reducing individual susceptibility to promotional messages. The former approach is the focus of this chapter, while the latter is the focus of subsequent chapters.

Existing justifications for policy approaches to protect children from the harmful effects of food marketing stem from risk-based or rights-based perspectives. These arguments correspond to different desired outcomes related to altering the marketing environment and/or individuals' responses to this environment (Figure 4.1). *Risk-based* arguments assert that children need protection from unhealthy food marketing to prevent poor diets and diet-related disease. This risk is partly predicated on children's heightened vulnerability and susceptibility to marketing influence, including as a result of their relatively immature cognitive development.

Piagetian theory outlines age-specific stages in the development of cognition that correlate with processing of marketing messages [7]. This theory proposes that children less than 8 years of age have an impaired ability to interpret marketing messages critically as they lack the necessary cognitive skills and experience. In effect, children are unable to evaluate marketing and tend to accept this as

The PROBLEM
Frequent exposure to persuasive marketing for unhealthy foods and beverages

Potential SOLUTIONS
Option 1: Socio-environmental solutions *(upstream approach)*
Option 2: Behavioural solutions *(mid-stream approach)*

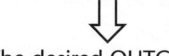

The desired OUTCOME
Option 1: Reduce <u>exposure</u> to, and <u>power</u> of, marketing *(reduce risks and protect rights)*
Option 2: Reduce <u>impact</u> on individuals *(reduce risks)*

FIGURE 4.1 Identifying policy solutions based on risk-based vs. rights-based arguments.

truthful, accurate and unbiased. However, more recent psychological theories (e.g. the Food Marketing Defense Model developed by Harris et al. [8]) suggest that understanding of marketing intent is a necessary but not a sufficient condition for decreasing individuals' vulnerability to marketing. One also needs the ability to produce counterarguments against marketing, and the motivation to do so [8]. As such, vulnerability to marketing extends beyond young childhood into adolescence, young adulthood and beyond. Researchers have argued that older adolescents and young adults also require protection from unhealthy food marketing [9]. Their unique vulnerability stems from their stage of identify formation and increased susceptibility to peer pressure, which is exploited by marketing that uses emotional appeals and which confers peer group social norms and expectations [8].

Alternatively, human *rights-based* arguments recognise the right for children to grow up without being undermined by corporate interests. As detailed in Chapter 3 of this book, unhealthy food marketing to children imposes on a number of rights protected under the United Nations' *Convention on the Rights of the Child* (1990). This includes the right to the enjoyment of the highest attainable standard of health, the right to adequate food and the right to privacy. The right to health extends the obligation of states to the provision of appropriate preventive and health promotion services, and children's *'right to grow and develop to their full potential and live in conditions that enable them to attain the highest standard of health through the implementation of programmes that address the underlying determinants of health'* [10]. Given the unequivocal evidence that children's exposure to unhealthy food marketing is a determinant of childhood unhealthy weight gain, preventive policy interventions to restrict this marketing are an obligation of states under the Convention [11]. The Convention also states that: *'Children have the right to reliable information from the media. Mass media such as television, radio and newspapers should provide information that children can understand and should not promote materials that could harm children* [Article 17]'. This argument has been adopted in some countries and territories, such as Sweden, Norway and Quebec, Canada, where all marketing to children (not only for food and beverages) is restricted on all or selected media.

Figure 4.1 integrates the two possible policy approaches – upstream and midstream – with risk-based and rights-based arguments for protecting children from the harmful effect of unhealthy food marketing. Only upstream policy interventions have the potential to address the risks associated with unhealthy food marketing exposures *and* ensure children's rights are protected from information and material that may be injurious to their well-being. Mid-stream policy approaches, in the absence of broader changes to the food marketing environment, may reduce the risks associated with food marketing exposures but do not act on the marketing environment itself. Behavioural approaches offer some potential to protect children in jurisdictions where food marketing restrictions are not presently viable, often due to government heeding strong private-sector opposition to regulation.

As such, mid-stream policy approaches may be expedient for reducing food marketing risks, while efforts are made to progress the political palatability of food marketing restrictions.

Global guidance on effective regulatory actions

To support upstream regulatory controls, in 2010 the World Health Organization released a set of recommendations to guide countries in developing or strengthening regulations to protect children from the harmful effects of food marketing [2]. The policy objective as stated in these recommendations was to restrict children's exposure to unhealthy food marketing and its power to impact on diet. That is, the recommendations apply a socio-environmental approach to protect children. The recommendations emphasise the important leadership role of governments in policy implementation and evaluation. A range of approaches are identified as possible, including both comprehensive restrictions that apply across all media and techniques, or stepwise restrictions that start by restricting selected media and/or techniques, with the aim of broadening restrictions over time. However, the recommendations identify that comprehensive approaches are likely to have the greatest impact. The recommendations were endorsed by all 193 member states of the World Health Assembly (resolution WHA63.14) [12]. Since this time, various implementation tools and reports have been prepared by the World Health Organization and its regional offices to support governments to implement the recommendations. This includes a *Framework for Implementing the Set of Recommendations* [3] and regional policy progress reports and recommendations for future action [11, 13].

The reality

Industry-led self-regulation of food marketing

Despite guidance from the World Health Organization on the need for regulations to protect children from unhealthy food marketing to be government-led, the predominant response to this issue globally has been the implementation of self-regulatory codes of practice, developed and enforced by the food and advertising industries [11, 13, 14]. Such codes may reflect good corporate responsibility, but, more likely, are a means of diverting industry criticism and impeding government regulations. The many limitations of existing food industry codes of practice for responsible food marketing to children suggest that they are not designed to be effective.

There are multiple factors that contribute to the ineffectiveness of industry self-regulatory codes for restricting food marketing to children. This includes their voluntary adoption, permissive nutrient criteria on which to base foods deemed acceptable to be promoted, and inadequate or vague definitions for when and where food marketing to children can occur [15, 16]. Industry pledges narrowly focus on food advertising 'directed to children' rather than considering the broader array of marketing to which children are exposed. Whether an advertisement is directed to children is determined by either the placement of the advertisement or its content, based on its themes, visuals or language. This means that, for the regulations to apply, an advertisement must be placed within a medium that is directed primarily to children (e.g. a children's television programme) or contain content that is primarily of appeal to children, and not also of main appeal to adolescents, parents or other adults. Critical reviews of self-regulatory codes demonstrate the ruse of such definitions. In Australia, for example, complaints to the Advertising Standards Panel about a Facebook and YouTube Cadbury Oreo chocolate advertisement, which featured an animated cartoon about a piece of chocolate playing with an Oreo biscuit at the beach, at a sports event and camping, and displaying emoticons that become happy when the pair unite, was not upheld because the themes in the advertisement were thought to elicit 'a whimsical feel of nostalgia' for adults and because the product was not a children's product but was designed for family sharing [17]. In Australia, three food and advertising industry codes of practice apply to food marketing to children – one from the grocery sector, one from the fast-food industry and one from the advertising industry. The Advertising Standards Panel makes determinations about breaches to these self-regulatory marketing codes of practice. All of these codes apply only to advertising 'directed to children' and few advertisements have been found to meet these criteria based on advertising content.

At the global level, the International Food & Beverage Alliance (IFBA) was established in 2008 and made a pledge to market food responsibly to children under 12 years of age [18]. This coincided with a call from the World Health Assembly in 2007 for a set of recommendations for member states on marketing of foods and beverages to children and pre-empted ensuing country actions. The IFBA pledge was most recently updated in 2014. Major limitations in the membership and scope of this pledge are evident, which preclude it from achieving the objectives stated in the World Health Organization recommendations for protecting children from the harmful effects of food marketing. At the time of writing (January, 2019), only 11 companies had signed up to the pledge, with many major food manufacturers, retailers and food service outlets/restaurants having not committed. Even for those companies that had committed to the pledge, the narrow scope of media, promotional techniques and foods covered by the restrictions serves to render the pledge ineffective. Major gaps in the scope of the IFBA pledge include:

1) *Media covered*: the pledge excludes packaging, in-store and point-of-sale marketing, and all forms of marketing communications that are not under the direct control of the company, such as online user-generated content (which often originates from food companies and is then shared virally). No mention is made of sponsorship of children's activities or marketing in settings where children gather.

2) *Persuasive techniques covered*: the pledge explicitly excludes brand equity characters, even though such characters are frequently used to promote unhealthy food to children and have been shown to influence children's food choices [19]. These are characters developed by a food company to be a mascot for a food brand.

3) *Narrow definition of when restrictions apply*: for example, restrictions to television advertising only apply during programmes for which at least 35% of the audience is under 12 years old. Television audience data show that in most countries this threshold is almost never achieved. Further, most of the television children watch is outside the confines of designated children's programmes and occurs during family viewing times.

4) *Narrow range of foods to which restrictions apply*: the pledge commits to market only products '*meeting specific nutrition criteria based on accepted scientific evidence and/or applicable national and international dietary guidelines*'. In practice, each signatory company determines its own nutritional criteria, which is typically set to be sympathetic to the company's product portfolio.

5) *Narrow age definition of a 'child'*: the pledge only applies to children under the age of 12 years. This is despite the growing and significant body of research suggesting that older children and even young adults are also negatively influenced by unhealthy food marketing [20].

In Europe, the food and beverage industries have introduced the EU Pledge, a similar self-regulatory code for marketing to children [21]. As with the IFBA pledge, signatory companies have committed not to advertise food on mass media where children under 12 years make up at least 35% of the audience, unless their products comply with nutrition criteria for 'healthier' products. As such, the same limitations and potential loopholes apply to this regional pledge as to the global commitment stated above.

Globally, variations in industry commitments across countries exist, despite most food marketing deriving from multinational corporations that advertise in all or most markets [22]. Typically, industry self-regulatory codes for responsible food marketing to children tend to operate in countries where there has been civil society pressure for government intervention. For example, in Australia vigorous public debate has occurred regarding if and how restrictions to children's exposure to unhealthy food marketing should occur, with civil society groups calling for government regulation [23]. Coinciding with this public debate, the food and advertising industries introduced multiple self-regulatory codes of practice for responsible food marketing to children. Meanwhile, in other countries without such vociferous public concern, no policies exist. This suggests that the primary motivation of the food industry in introducing self-regulatory measures is to stall and interfere with government regulation, rather than to reduce children's exposure to unhealthy food marketing and its power. This is unsurprising, given that food companies' primary responsibility is to their shareholders to increase profits and marketing is one of the most effective tools to leverage product sales.

Evaluations of industry self-regulatory approaches for responsible food marketing indicate that, to date, these have had minimal or no effect in reducing children's exposures to unhealthy food marketing. Paradoxically, research has found that signatories to industry's responsible advertising codes often promote unhealthy foods at higher rates than non-signatory companies [24]. In Canada, for example, analysis of television broadcasting across two provinces (Ontario and Quebec) in 2011 found that companies that were signatories to the Canadian Children's Food and Beverage Initiative were responsible for significantly more food advertisements than non-signatory companies during children's preferred viewing times and the nutritional quality of foods promoted by signatories was poorer, being higher in fats, sugar, sodium and energy [25].

Comparing across countries, other research has found that countries with industry self-regulation appear to have higher rates of unhealthy food advertising than those countries that do not have any existing policies regulation to restrict children's exposures to this marketing. One study compared television food advertising rates across 22 countries with different policy arrangements, including government regulations, industry self-regulations or no regulations [22]. During children's peak viewing times, defined as the top five 1-hour timeslots for weekdays and weekend days in each country, the rate of advertising for unhealthy foods was significantly higher in countries that had industry self-regulatory codes of practice for responsible food marketing to children compared to those countries with no policies at all. In countries with industry regulation, there was an average of 3.8 unhealthy food advertisements per hour, compared to 2.6 advertisements per hour in countries with no policy [22]. While this difference is ostensibly small, if children watched 2 hours of television per day during these peak viewing times this would equate to 730 more unhealthy food advertisement exposures over a year, equivalent to an additional 6 hours of unhealthy food advertising given most advertisements are approximately 30 seconds in duration.

Government-led regulation of food marketing

Globally, governments in a number of countries have introduced statutory regulation to protect children from unhealthy food marketing, either across all media or on selected media. The World Cancer Research Fund maintains a database of policies that have been implemented in countries across the world to promote healthy diets and reduce obesity, called the NOURISHING database [26]. This includes policies to restrict unhealthy food marketing to children. As at the end of 2018, four jurisdictions had introduced comprehensive government regulations on unhealthy food marketing to children that applied across all media and settings. This included Brazil, Finland, Peru and Quebec, Canada. A greater number of countries had introduced food marketing restrictions on broadcast media only, including television and/or radio, including Chile, Iran, Ireland, Mexico, Norway, South Korea, Sweden, Taiwan, Turkey and the UK.

Government-led food marketing regulations vary in terms of the nutritional values of products restricted, marketing media covered, restrictions to marketing techniques and penalties (if any) for non-compliance. In many cases, restrictions apply to marketing 'directed to children' as defined by the proportion of children in the audience and/or by the use of techniques that would appeal to children, such as animations and toys. With the use of such definitions, it is relatively straightforward for marketers to circumvent the spirit of the regulations while upholding the letter of the law. For example, marketing campaigns may be modified to use themes that appeal to older children or adolescents not covered by the regulations, or to be shown on media that attract high numbers of older users or viewers as well as children. As such, children's actual exposures to unhealthy food marketing may remain unchanged despite their exposure to 'child-directed' marketing having decreased.

This was identified to be the case in the UK following the introduction of government-led regulations to restrict unhealthy food and beverage advertising on television. The UK regulations restrict unhealthy food advertising on dedicated children's channels and during programmes that attract a high *proportion* of child viewers relative to adults. This represents a significant potential loophole in the regulations whereby food advertising in popular family programmes can continue unabated. For example, if a prime-time programme attracted three million viewers and 15% of these were children (450,000), this programme would not be covered by the regulations. However, if a child-directed cartoon programme attracted 600,000 viewers and 30% of these were children (180,000), this would be covered. Evaluations of changes to children and adults' exposures to unhealthy television food advertising after the introduction of the regulations identified that exposures increased for all population groups, including children, given that advertising shifted from the lesser-watched children's television programmes to family programmes that enjoyed higher absolute numbers of child viewers [27].

Such evaluations of the outcomes of regulatory interventions are important for identifying if the policy is having the intended effect and whether any unintended consequences occur. Despite the growing number of countries that have introduced government regulations to protect children from the harmful effects of unhealthy food marketing, relatively few studies are available in the public domain to evaluate the impact of these regulations on children's marketing exposures or children's responses to food marketing, including their food preferences, purchases, consumption or body weight. The following section provides an account of the major findings of available evaluations of government-led food marketing regulations.

Impact of regulations on children's food marketing exposures

Two systematic reviews of the scientific evidence have examined the literature on the effectiveness of government statutory regulations on food marketing [24, 28]. From these reviews, most studies have found that statutory regulations had produced successful outcomes in relation to reducing children's exposure to unhealthy food marketing, particularly on television (to which most regulations apply). For example, in South Korea, the Special Act on Safety Management of Children's Dietary Life restricts unhealthy food marketing on television between 5 and 7 p.m. and during children's programmes starting from September 2010. Evaluation of this Act identified that, following its implementation, the total advertising expenditure, number of advertisement placements and child gross rating points (audience size) for unhealthy foods decreased during the regulated hours [29]. Comparing 4 months before the introduction of the regulations to 4 months after their introduction, the number of unhealthy food advertisements dropped by 81% during regulated hours with a commensurate drop in advertising expenditure. Promisingly, advertising budgets for healthier products increased following the introduction of the regulation, such that the overall advertising budget for all foods increased by 13% despite a relative drop in advertising expenditure for unhealthy products. This suggests the possibility for replacement advertising to fill the void that removing unhealthy food advertisements would create. This is a potentially important point to assuage arguments that the quality of children's programming would be diminished should broadcasters' revenue be reduced. It also opens opportunities for the promotion of healthier food products, which may have positive impacts on food knowledge and behaviours, as outlined in the last part of this book.

Reductions in children's exposures to unhealthy food marketing as a result of government-led regulations have been found to exceed that of any changes in countries with industry self-regulation or no regulations for responsible marketing [24, 28]. However, limitations to the regulations have tempered their effectiveness. For example, restrictions to advertisement length in the USA had led to a greater number of total advertisements of shorter duration. In Quebec, Canada, restrictions only apply to broadcasting originating from that province, meaning that English-language television channels that come from other provinces and the USA remain unregulated. Evaluations of the Quebecois regulation find that Quebec French-speaking children were exposed to less unhealthy food marketing. However, Quebec English-speaking children were still exposed to high levels of unhealthy food marketing [30, 31]. While the Quebec regulations also extend online, an evaluation of food and restaurant company websites found there to be no difference in the presence of child-directed content, such as 'advergames' (branded online games) and branded downloadable items, between French-language websites and English-language websites [32].

French-language websites were covered under Quebec's Consumer Protection Act of 1978, while the English-language websites were not covered. Quebec's Consumer Protection Act relies on public complaints to identify breaches rather than active monitoring of compliance. This may limit the extent of implementation of the regulations, particularly for new media where the public may be less aware of the regulatory remit and for which the public (parents) may be less aware of what children are exposed to and so would be less inclined to complain about a potential breach.

As noted above, in the UK, evaluations have shown that unhealthy television food advertising rates reduced in children's television programming after the introduction of regulations [27]. However, there was no change in children's overall exposures to unhealthy food advertising as the rate of this advertising increased during other broadcast times, which still corresponded to large numbers of child viewers but also high adult viewership. Comparing television advertising data between 2010 after full implementation of the UK regulations to 2008, which corresponded to part-implementation of the regulations, there was a slight increase in the proportion of food advertisements that were for unhealthy foods during children's peak viewing times at follow-up. That is, when the greatest numbers of children were viewing. Importantly, these peak viewing times did not necessarily correspond with regulated broadcast times, given restrictions were based on the proportion of child viewers rather than actual viewing numbers.

Impact of regulations on children's food marketing responses

Only limited evidence is available to evaluate the impact of government regulations on children's responses to food marketing. No studies are available to assess the impact of restrictions on children's food preferences, food choices, dietary intakes or health outcomes. This is perhaps unsurprising, given that even if television advertising was effectively regulated, children would still be exposed to food marketing through a raft of other avenues. Effects of marketing restrictions on body weight would also only be seen over time and not as an imminent outcome of any one policy, no matter how well designed that policy were. However, a small number of studies have quantified the impact of regulations on food purchases or sales, thereby showing the great importance of installing effective regulations for food marketing [33, 34]. Others have estimated the potential impact of regulations on children's body weight status using data modelling and simulation (for example, [35]).

One recent study compared the sales of unhealthy food items over time across countries that had implemented broadcast marketing policies, including statutory regulations and industry self-regulation [33]. Those countries with statutory regulations saw, on average, a statistically significant 9% decrease in unhealthy food sales per capita after the introduction of the regulations. Alternatively, in those countries where only self-regulation had been implemented, sales of unhealthy foods per capita significantly increased by 2%.

In the UK, a study evaluated the impact of the UK Government food advertising restrictions on household purchases of unhealthy foods using the UK Living Costs and Food Survey; a continuous annual survey of household expenditures commissioned by the UK Government [34]. Following the intro-duction of statutory regulation to restrict unhealthy food advertising to children on television, households with children increased their fruit and vegetable expenditure per capita by £5.00 per quarter and decreased their expenditure on unhealthy foods and beverages by £8.90 per capita per quarter. A similar change in unhealthy food and beverage expenditure was also observed following the earlier introduction of industry self-regulation, as compared to household expenditures when no regulation was in place. However, only statutory regu-lation led to a reduction in television advertising expenditures and thus food advertising exposures [34].

A similar, earlier, study from Canada used Canadian household expenditure data to evaluate the impact of Quebec's Consumer Protection Act on purchases of fast food [36]. The study compared French-speaking and English-speaking households across two provinces – Quebec, with food marketing restrictions, and Ontario, without food marketing restrictions. Changes to fast-food purchases following the introduction of the Consumer Protection Act were identified in expected direc-tions. That is, French-speaking households with children living in Quebec were less likely to buy fast food than English-speaking households in Quebec, recalling that English-speaking children from Quebec had greater access to media from outside the province and were therefore less impacted by the marketing restrictions. The findings were not an artefact of cultural variances in fast food purchases, with no changes in purchasing behaviours over time in French-speaking households com-pared to English-speaking households in Ontario. Overall, there was a 13% decrease in the purchase propensity (likelihood to buy) fast food for French-speaking house-holds in Quebec. These examples make clear that similar and parallel regulations should be implemented in order to improve eating behaviour among all children in a certain region.

Lastly, multiple studies have simulated with econometric analyses the likely effect of food marketing regulations on children's weight status and thus obesity-related diseases and health care costs [35, 37–39]. These studies suggest that regulation to restrict children's exposures to unhealthy food advertising on television would be a cost-saving intervention [37–39], with the greatest ben-efits accrued by children living in the most disadvantaged areas who are known to watch more television (in Australia, the study country) [35]. Estimates from these studies have been based on evidence from experimental trials of the impact of food marketing exposures on children, rather than evaluations of real-world implementation of food marketing restrictions, for which there is a lack of robust data.

The role of stakeholders in building effective solutions

Campaigning for the protection of children from unhealthy food marketing may appear an insurmountable challenge, given the economic power and influence of the food and beverage manufacturing, retail and service industries. This is a hugely concentrated and powerful industry [40]. Global advertising data show that the top ten advertising companies contribute to 40% of all unhealthy food advertisements on television across markets [22]. Nevertheless, there is now a resonant global policy mandate that calls for the introduction of government-led regulations to restrict children's exposure to unhealthy food marketing [2] and this has been agreed upon unilaterally by governments across the world through the World Health Assembly (resolution WHA61.14). There is also a growing evidence base detailing 'what works' and, importantly, 'what does not work' for regulations to protect children. Despite this, moving towards this policy agenda will require political impetus for action, brought about by robust and convincing evidence on the need to act and an engaged civil society to hold elected politicians to account.

Academia, civil society and professional health associations can act as catalysts for change and counterbalance the strong opposition from the food and advertising industries on government-led regulations to restrict children's exposures to unhealthy food marketing. Case examples from Latin American countries highlight how research and policy advocacy by civil society and academia supported the introduction of some of the most pioneering food environment regulations globally, including relating to food marketing to children [41]. These regulations were underpinned by the generation of local-level research to highlight the scope of the issue and its solutions. Critically, this research informed evidence-based advocacy and public education spurred through multi-sectoral coalitions to advance public awareness and concern about the issue and apply political pressure to act [41].

Conclusion

Considering the evidence overall, it is reasonable to conclude that, to date, industry self-regulation of unhealthy food marketing to children has had more value as corporate spin than actual merit in reducing children's exposures to unhealthy food marketing. Government-led regulations hold more promise, and at a global level there is some evidence that these regulations have reduced children's exposures to unhealthy food marketing, with subsequent reductions in the sale or purchase of unhealthy foods and beverages. However, the details of the regulations are crucially important to ensure their success and prevent circumvention by industry, and the shifting of marketing budgets to less-regulated media and techniques. All of society has a stake in this issue to ensure that children can achieve the highest attainable health. Equally, all of society has a role in progressing effective solutions, including through political activism and advocating for social change.

References

1 World Health Organization Western Pacific Region. *WHO nutrient profile model for the Western Pacific Region*. 2016 [accessed 8 October 2018]; Available from: http://apps.who.int/iris/bitstream/handle/10665/252082/9789290617853-eng.pdf;jsessionid=BC4D4CEA04232CE8675BC08900662400?sequence=1.

2 World Health Organization. *Set of recommendations on the marketing of foods and non-alcoholic beverages to children*. 2010 [accessed 15 October 2018]; Available from: www.who.int/dietphysicalactivity/marketing-food-to-children/en/.

3 World Health Organization. *A framework for implementing the set of recommendations on the marketing of foods and non-alcoholic beverages to children*. 2012 [accessed 8 October 2018]; Available from: http://www.who.int/dietphysicalactivity/MarketingFramework2012.pdf?ua=1.

4 Keller, K.L. Unlocking the power of integrated marketing communications: How integrated is your IMC program? *Journal of Advertising*, 2016. **45**(3): 286–301.

5 World Health Organization. *Set of recommendations on the marketing of foods and non-alcoholic beverages to children*. 2010, WHO: Geneva.

6 Sacks, G., B. Swinburn, and M. Lawrence. Obesity policy action framework and analysis grids for a comprehensive policy approach to reducing obesity. *Obesity Reviews*, 2009. **10**(1): 76–86.

7 Calvert, S.L. Children as consumers: Advertising and marketing. *The Future of Children*, 2008. **18**(1): 205–234.

8 Harris, J.L., K.D. Brownell, and J.A. Bargh. The Food Marketing Defense Model: Integrating psychological research to protect youth and inform public policy. *Social Issues and Policy Review*, 2009. **3**(1): 211–271.

9 Freeman, B., et al. Young adults: Beloved by food and drink marketers and forgotten by public health? *Health Promotion International*, 2016. **31**(4): 954–961.

10 Committee on the Rights of the Child. *General comment no. 15 (2013) on the right of the child to the enjoyment of the highest attainable standard of health (Article 24)*. 2013 [accessed 8 January 2019]; Available from: http://docstore.ohchr.org/SelfServices/FilesHandler.ashx?enc=6QkG1d%2FPPRiCAqhKb7yhsqIkirKQZLK2M58RF%2F5F0vHCIs1B9k1r3x0aA7FYrehlNUfw4dHmlOxmFtmhaiMOkH80ywS3uq6Q3bqZ3A3yQ0%2B4u6214CSatnrBlZT8nZmj.

11 World Health Organization Regional Office for Europe. *Evaluating implementation of the WHO set of recommendations on the marketing of foods and non-alcoholic beverages to children. Progress, challenges and guidance for next steps in the WHO European region* 2018; Available from: http://www.euro.who.int/__data/assets/pdf_file/0003/384015/food-marketing-kids-eng.pdf?ua=1.

12 World Health Assembly. *Marketing of food and non-alcoholic beverages to children*, in *WHA63.14*. 2010, WHO: Geneva.

13 World Health Organization. Regional Office for the Eastern Mediterranean. *Implementing the WHO recommendations on the marketing of food and non-alcoholic beverages to children in the Eastern Mediterranean Region*. 2018, WHO Regional Office for the Eastern Mediterranean: Cairo.

14 Kraak, V.I., et al. Progress achieved in restricting the marketing of high-fat, sugary and salty food and beverage products to children. *Bulletin of the World Health Organization*, 2016. **94**(7): 540–548.

15 Hebden, L., et al., Industry self-regulation of food marketing to children: Reading the fine print. *Health Promotion Journal of Australia*, 2010. **21**: 229–235.

16 Ronit, K. and J.D. Jensen. Obesity and industry self-regulation of food and beverage marketing: A literature review. *European Journal of Clinical Nutrition*, 2014. **68**: 753.

17 Obesity Policy Coalition. *Overbranded, underprotected. How industry self-regulation is failing to protect children from unhealthy food marketing.* 2018 [accessed 8 January 2019]; Available from: http://www.opc.org.au/downloads/overbranded/overbranded-under-protected.pdf.

18 International Food & Beverage Alliance. *Our commitments: Responsible marketing to children.* 2014 [accessed 29 October 2018]; Available from: https://www.ifballiance.org/uploads/media/59eddc9fba341.pdf.

19 McGale, L., et al. The influence of brand equity characters on children's food preferences and choices. *Journal of Pediatrics,* 2016. **177**: 33–38.

20 World Health Organization. Regional Office for Europe. *Tackling food marketing to children in a digital world: Trans-disciplinary perspectives. Children's rights, evidence of impact, methodological challenges, regulatory options and policy implications for the WHO European Region.* 2016 [accesed 15 October 2018]; Available from: http://www.euro.who.int/__data/assets/pdf_file/0017/322226/Tackling-food-marketing-children-digital-world-trans-disciplinary-perspectives-en.pdf.

21 World Federation of Advertisers. *EU Pledge* 2019 [accessed 11 March 2019]; Available from: http://www.eu-pledge.eu/.

22 Kelly B, et al. Global benchmarking of children's potential exposures to unhealthful food advertising on television. *Obesity Reviews,* in press.

23 Hebden, L., et al. Industry self-regulation of food marketing to children: Reading the fine print. *Health Promotion Journal of Australia,* 2010. **21**(3): 229–235.

24 Galbraith-Emami, S. and T. Lobstein. The impact of initiatives to limit the advertising of food and beverage products to children: A systematic review. *Obesity Reviews,* 2013. **14**(12): 960–974.

25 Potvin Kent, M., L. Dubois, and A. Wanless. Self regulation by industry in food marketing is having little impact during children's preferred television viewing. *Canadian Journal of Diabetes,* 2011. **35**(2): 151.

26 World Cancer Research Fund. *NOURISHING database.* 2018 [accessed 18 December 2018]; Available from: https://www.wcrf.org/int/policy/nourishing-database.

27 Adams, J., et al. Effect of restrictions on television food advertising to children on exposure to advertisements for 'less healthy' foods: Repeat cross-sectional study. *PloS One,* 2012. **7**(2): e31578–e31578.

28 Chambers, S.A., et al. Reducing the volume, exposure and negative impacts of advertising for foods high in fat, sugar and salt to children: A systematic review of the evidence from statutory and self-regulatory actions and educational measures. *Preventive Medicine,* 2015. **75**: 32–43.

29 Kim, S., et al. Restriction of television food advertising in South Korea: Impact on advertising of food companies. *Health Promotion International,* 2013. **28**(1): 17–25.

30 Potvin Kent, M., L. Dubois, and A. Wanless. Food marketing on children's television in two different policy environments. *International Journal of Pediatric Obesity,* 2011. **6**(suppl. 3): e433–e441.

31 Potvin Kent, M., L. Dubois, and A. Wanless. A nutritional comparison of foods and beverages marketed to children in two advertising policy environments. *Obesity (Silver Spring),* 2012. **20**(9): 1829–1837.

32 Potvin Kent, M., et al. Internet marketing directed at children on food and restaurant websites in two policy environments. *Obesity,* 2013. **21**(4): 800–807.

33 Kovic, Y., et al. The impact of junk food marketing regulations on food sales: an ecological study. *Obesity Reviews,* 2018. **19**(6): 761–769.

34 Silva, A., L.M. Higgins, and M. Hussein. An evaluation of the effect of child-directed television food advertising regulation in the United Kingdom. *Canadian Journal of Agricultural Economics/Revue canadienne d'agroeconomie*, 2015. **63**(4): 583–600.

35 Brown, V., et al. The potential cost-effectiveness and equity impacts of restricting television advertising of unhealthy food and beverages to Australian children. *Nutrients*, 2018. **10**(5): 622.

36 Dhar, T. and K. Baylis. Fast-food consumption and the ban on advertising targeting children: The Quebec experience. *Journal of Marketing Research (JMR)*, 2011. **48**(5): 799–813.

37 Magnus, A., et al. The cost-effectiveness of removing television advertising of high-fat and/or high-sugar food and beverages to Australian children. *International Journal of Obesity*, 2009. **33**: 1094.

38 Sonneville, K.R., et al. BMI and healthcare cost impact of eliminating tax subsidy for advertising unhealthy food to youth. *American Journal of Preventive Medicine*, 2015. **49**(1): 124–134.

39 Cecchini, M., et al. Tackling of unhealthy diets, physical inactivity, and obesity: Health effects and cost-effectiveness. *The Lancet*, 2010. **376**(9754): 1775–1784.

40 Oxfam. *Behind the brands. Food justice and the 'Big 10' food and beverage companies*. 2013 [accessed 8 January 2019]; Available from: https://www.oxfam.org/sites/www.oxfam.org/files/bp166-behind-the-brands-260213-en.pdf.

41 Pérez-Escamilla, R., et al. Prevention of childhood obesity and food policies in Latin America: From research to practice. *Obesity Reviews*, 2017. **18**(S2): 28–38.

5

IMPROVING ADVERTISING LITERACY AND EFFECTIVENESS

Dr. Esther Rozendaal

A large body of research has investigated children's susceptibility to the persuasive appeal of food advertising. These studies convincingly showed that advertising – in all its shapes and sizes – stimulates children's awareness of and desire for advertised food products and brands, their food purchase requests to parents and their own food purchase behavior (e.g., Buijzen & Valkenburg, 2003; D'Alessio, Laghi, & Baiocco, 2009; Valkenburg & Buijzen, 2005). Moreover, research has also evidenced that these so-called "intended" effects of advertising may lead to certain "unintended," and often undesired, consequences for children's wellbeing, such as parent–child conflict and unhealthy eating habits (e.g., Boyland & Whalen, 2015; Buijzen & Valkenburg, 2003; Roberts & Pettigrew, 2013).

Besides concerns over the negative effects of food advertising on the wellbeing of children, there are also concerns about the honesty of food advertising directly targeting children. In comparison with adults, children are thought to be more vulnerable to food advertising and, as a consequence, more susceptible to its impact. The rationale behind this assumption is that children's advertising literacy (i.e., understanding of the commercial nature of and persuasive tactics used in advertising) has not fully developed yet, and that therefore they are less capable of evaluating advertising in general, and food advertising in specific, in a critical manner (Harris, Brownell, & Bargh, 2009; Rozendaal, Lapierre, Van Reijmersdal, & Buijzen, 2011). These issues of fairness are even more severe in the contemporary media environment, which is characterized by subtle advertising formats that are integrated in entertainment. Children have great difficulty recognizing the commercial nature of these practices (De Jans, Van de Sompel, Hudders, & Cauberghe, 2017).

As a result of these concerns, there is an increasing call for restrictive regulations to protect children from food advertising. However, the global nature of contemporary digital advertising makes it increasingly difficult to implement and control restrictive advertising policies. Moreover, as food advertising involves major financial interests, the implementation of restrictive regulations has little support among manufacturers and advertisers and is therefore complex and often not effective. As an alternative, many countries therefore focus on the empowerment of children as critical consumers through advertising literacy education (e.g., www.mediasmart.uk.com; www.consumer.ftc.gov/admongo).

In this chapter I will discuss the conceptualization of advertising literacy, how children's advertising literacy develops with age, the role of advertising literacy in children's susceptibility to food advertising, and how media education and sponsorship disclosures can increase children's advertising literacy skills in order to empower them to cope with food advertising.

Conceptualization of advertising literacy

In the children and advertising literature, advertising literacy has mainly been approached from a cognitive perspective (for an overview, see Wright, Friestad, & Boush, 2005). At least seven cognitive components of advertising literacy have been identified, varying from very simple to more complex and abstract types of knowledge (Rozendaal et al., 2011):

1. recognition of advertising – differentiating advertising from other media content;
2. recognition of advertising's source – understanding who pays for advertising messages;
3. perception of intended audience – understanding the concept of audience targeting and segmentation;
4. understanding advertising's selling intent – understanding that advertising tries to sell products;
5. understanding advertising's persuasive intent – understanding that advertising attempts to influence consumers' behavior by changing their mental states;
6. understanding advertisers' persuasive tactics – understanding specific persuasion strategies used by advertisers;
7. understanding advertising's bias – being aware of discrepancies between the advertised and the actual product.

However, over the years, many advertising literacy scholars have argued that this cognitive focus on advertising literacy might be too narrow a conceptualization. According to these scholars (Hudders et al., 2017; Rozendaal et al., 2011), the concept of advertising literacy should not only entail the ability to identify and understand advertising messages, but also the ability to cope with those messages critically. Therefore, Rozendaal et al. (2011) proposed another dimension of advertising literacy, which they refer to as attitudinal advertising literacy. Attitudinal advertising literacy consists of two components that should be added to the traditional conceptualization of advertising literacy:

1. skepticism toward advertising – the tendency toward disbelief of advertising;
2. disliking of advertising – a general negative attitude toward advertising.

Along with attitudinal advertising literacy, Rozendaal et al. (2011) also introduced a third dimension of advertising literacy: advertising literacy performance. As will become apparent in the remainder of the chapter, children who have the necessary conceptual and attitudinal advertising literacy in place do not necessarily retrieve this literacy when confronted with advertising and apply it as a critical defense (Brucks, Armstrong, & Goldberg, 1988; Rozendaal, Buijzen, & Valkenburg, 2012). Therefore, Rozendaal et al (2011) argued that the theoretical distinction between conceptual and attitudinal advertising literacy (i.e., having advertising knowledge and holding a general critical attitude towards it) and advertising literacy performance (i.e., retrieving and applying advertising knowledge and attitudes when confronted with advertising) should be emphasized more strongly in conceptualizing advertising literacy. The advertising literacy performance dimension comprises two components:

1. retrieval of advertising literacy – the ability to retrieve relevant advertising-related knowledge and attitudes from memory while processing an advertising message;
2. application of advertising literacy – the ability to apply advertising-related knowledge and attitudes to an advertising message while processing the message.

Recently, Hudders et al. (2017) extended Rozendaal's three-dimensional conceptualization of advertising literacy with an additional dimension: moral advertising literacy. Moral advertising literacy reflects individuals' ability to develop thoughts about the moral appropriateness of specific advertising formats and comprises the general moral evaluations individuals hold toward these formats (e.g., advergames, brand placement, or TV commercials) and toward advertising in general, including its persuasive tactics (e.g., humor or celebrity endorsements, using personal data to customize commercial messages). This dimension is deeply intertwined with the ability to notice when advertising is biased (e.g., one-sided or misleading) and the tendency toward disbelief of advertising.

The development of children's advertising literacy

An extensive and long-established body of research has focused on the development of children's advertising literacy (for reviews, see De Jans, Van de Sompel et al., 2017; John, 1999; Kunkel et al., 2004, Wright et al., 2005). Most of these studies have concentrated on two of advertising literacy's cognitive or conceptual components: recognition of advertising and understanding of its intent. Recognition of advertising is generally defined as the ability to distinguish commercial content from non-commercial content. For example, it has been shown that before about 5 years of age, children still have great difficulty distinguishing commercials from television programs and, thus, view advertising primarily as entertainment. However, around the age of 7, the majority of children are able to recognize the difference between television advertising and programs. Yet, in comparison with television commercials, children find it far more difficult to recognize digital advertising formats, such as brand placements in games, as a form of persuasion. The most significant explanation for this is that these forms of advertising are integrated into editorial content (e.g., on a website) or entertainment (e.g., in a game or a television program), whereas this is not the case with traditional television commercials. An advertising banner on a website is on the computer screen at the same time as the editorial content of that website. In games, the commercial message is in general entirely woven into the game itself, such as advergames. There are, therefore, far fewer identifiable commercial characteristics, and consequently, children find it much more difficult to recognize these forms of advertising.

Around the age of 8, children demonstrate an increasing understanding of the intent of advertising. Studies have consistently shown that more than three-quarters of all children understand the selling intent of traditional television commercials around the age of 8 (for reviews, see Hudders et al., 2017; John, 1999; Kunkel et al., 2004). From this age onwards, children understand that commercials are not shown on television as a toilet break, but that they are designed to advertise and sell products. This insight develops further as children get older. Around the age of 11 children understand that advertisers are trying to persuade them to buy a certain brand or product by influencing their thoughts and opinions about that brand or product. They also increasingly gain insight into the tactics that are deployed by advertisers to tempt them and others (Rozendaal et al., 2012). What these studies show is that children develop the understanding of the persuasive intent of television commercials noticeably later than the understanding of its selling intent. This is in line with Moses and Baldwin's (2005) assumption that it is easier for children to understand that advertisers try to change their behavior (i.e., selling intent) than to understand that they try to change their mental states (i.e., persuasive intent). That is, to understand the persuasive intent of advertising, children have to be empathetic and be able to put themselves into the position of advertisers, and apply their reasoning. This way of reasoning is necessary to make a link between the use of certain temptation techniques (for instance, "if an advertisement is very funny....") and a certain desired impact ("…. then the advertisers want me to like the advertisement"). From the age of 10, children are increasingly more capable of doing so.

In comparison with traditional television commercials children find it far more difficult to understand the commercial nature of most types of advertising in digital media, primarily because they don't recognize it as a commercial message due to its embedded and often actively involving nature (Nairn & Fine, 2008). Specifically, in digital media, advertising is embedded into non-promotional media content (e.g., entertainment, information). Embedding advertisements into non-promotional media content blurs the distinction between advertising, information, and media content (Calvert, 2008; Moore, 2004), which makes it more difficult for children to recognize the content as advertised content. This may be especially the case for less-experienced consumers, as children are. Furthermore, digital advertising formats are interactive in nature. Interactive advertising formats (e.g., advergames) are often challenging and motivate children to keep interacting, resulting in a longer length of brand exposure. The interactivity in itself demands cognitive capacity of children, which reduces the capacity to think about the nature of advertising messages, since individuals only have limited cognitive resources (cf. Limited Capacity Model; Lang, 2000).

A number of studies have indeed shown that children's recognition and understanding of embedded forms of advertising, such as brand placements in videos, in-game advertising, and advergames, develop considerably later than their understanding of television advertising (e.g., Auty & Lewis, 2004; Hudders, Cauberghe, & Panic, 2016; Mallinckrodt and Mizerski, 2007; Owen, Lewis, Auty, & Buijzen, 2013; Panic, Cauberghe, and De Pelsmacker, 2013; Rozendaal, Slot, van Reijmersdal, & Buijzen, 2013; Van Reijmersdal, Rozendaal, & Buijzen, 2012; Verhellen, Oates, De Pelsmacker, & Dens, 2014; Waiguny & Terlutter, 2011; Wollslager, 2009). For example, Owen and colleagues (2013) found that 6–10-year-old children showed a significantly less sophisticated understanding of the persuasive intent of brand placement in movies and games in comparison to television commercials. In addition, Van Reijmersdal et al. (2012) found that almost half of the 9–12-year-old children in their sample were not aware that food advergames are created by food companies (i.e., Lays and Pepsi) and did not understand that the game was intended to make them like the advertised food products. The study also showed that children's liking of advergames was high, suggesting that they did not hold a critical attitude toward it.

The role of advertising literacy in children's susceptibility to food advertising

In the societal and academic debate on the impact of unhealthy food advertising on children it is often assumed that advertising literacy makes children less susceptible to food advertising effects. The rationale underlying this assumption is the idea that the main defense against food advertising is a cognitive one and, therefore, knowledge on advertising's intent and tactics can function as a filter when processing food advertising messages. In this so-called cognitive defense view, children who possess the necessary knowledge of advertising will use this knowledge in order to critically process the ads they encounter, making them less susceptible to its effects, including advertised food product preferences and requests (e.g., Brucks et al., 1988; Friestad & Wright, 1994).

However, existing research does not provide convincing empirical evidence for the cognitive defense of children towards food advertising. Only few studies found that a better understanding of the persuasive nature of a food advertisement leads to less persuasion among children (e.g., less positive brand attitudes and lower advertised product desire; for an exception, see Waiguny, Nelson, & Terlutter, 2012). Most studies failed to demonstrate a direct effect of understanding the persuasive nature of advertisements (including food advertisements) on persuasion (for an overview, see Mizerski, Wang, Lee, & Lambert, 2017). Furthermore, research that uses age as a proxy for children's level of advertising literacy because the two are highly correlated does not provide clear evidence for the cognitive defense view either. In their comprehensive literature review, Livingstone and Helsper (2006) showed that the empirical evidence on the relationship between children's age and their responses to food advertising does not support the belief that older children, who are assumed to have higher levels of advertising literacy, are less susceptible to food advertising effects. In other words, there is little evidence to suggest that an increase in advertising literacy indeed leads to reduced food advertising effects.

A possible reason for the absence of a direct relationship between children's conceptual advertising literacy and their susceptibility to food advertising is that, even if we grant that children have the necessary conceptual knowledge about advertising in place, it does not necessarily follow that they will actually enact it as a critical defense against its persuasive appeal (Brucks et al., 1988; John, 1999; Moses & Baldwin, 2005). To defend against food advertising successfully, children need to engage in advertising coping strategies (e.g., formulate critical thoughts, activate avoidance strategies). However, insights on children's advertising processing (Buijzen, Van Reijmersdal, & Owen, 2010) and cognitive development (Moses & Baldwin, 2005) suggest that, due to the powerful emotional appeal of food advertising, combined with their immature cognitive abilities, children lack the motivation and ability to retrieve and apply their advertising-related knowledge while confronted with food advertising and choose a relevant coping strategy as a critical defense (i.e., advertising literacy performance; Rozendaal et al., 2011). Moreover, because of the highly involving nature of most advertised food products, and their evolutionary preference for food (especially foods high in salt, sugar, and fat), children's desire to conform to the message may be much stronger than their desire to defend against it (Harris et al., 2009).

Empowering children to cope with food advertising through advertising education

The increasing amount of food advertising children are faced with in today's media has led to a growing call for initiatives that can empower children to cope with food advertising and defend against its undesired effects. A way to empower children to critically cope with food advertising is through advertising literacy training, for example, through educational interventions in schools or by parents (Livingstone & Helsper, 2006). Over the past few years, a number of educational programs focusing on advertising have been implemented, varying from multiple-hour in-class curricula (e.g., www.mediasmart.uk.com; www.reclamewijs. mediawijs.be) to educational games (e.g., www.consumer.ftc.gov/admongo), and short training sessions as part of larger media literacy curricula (e.g., www.mediaeducationlab.com). In general, the purpose of these programs is to develop children's knowledge about the purpose and tactics of advertising, and to provide critical thinking skills and coping mechanisms in order to make better-educated decisions regarding the food products that are presented in the advertising.

Despite calls for research focusing on the development and testing of advertising education programs (Wright et al., 2005), scientific research is still scarce (see for an overview Jeong, Cho, & Hwang, 2012). The handful of studies conducted on advertising education effectiveness indeed showed that these programs can be effective in enhancing children's understanding of and critical attitudes toward advertising. For example, a field study by Nelson (2016) showed that just a few hours of training could result in significant increases in several aspects of advertising-related knowledge, including understanding of selling intent, understanding of persuasive tactics, and awareness of the commercial source and target audience. In addition, a study by Hudders et al. (2016) demonstrated that a short 15-minute training session in the classroom improved the children's understanding of the persuasive intent of advergames. However, this increased understanding did not decrease their desire for the advertised product when playing an advergame for the chocolate pudding brand Paula de Cow. In a comparable study, De Jans, Hudder, and Cauberghe (2017) showed that a short 10-minute advertising literacy training session can improve children's recognition and understanding of a product placement of the brand M&M's in the movie *The Smurfs*. They also found that this increased cognitive advertising literacy had an influence on the effectiveness of product placement (i.e., purchase request) when children's general ad liking was low, though not when it was high.

This research shows that, as has been argued before in this chapter, having higher levels of advertising knowledge does not automatically enable children to defend against food advertising. In other words, knowledge on the persuasive intent and tactics of food advertising does not automatically result in increased critical processing of the advertisement or resistance towards the advertised food products. Therefore, educational advertising interventions that focus primarily on increasing children's understanding of food advertising's intent and persuasive tactics are unlikely to be effective in empowering children to defend against food advertising. Having knowledge of advertising is a necessary precondition for children to defend against advertising, because it is only when they are able to recognize a message as a form of advertising that they will have the opportunity to defend against it. However, to cope with food advertising successfully, children also need to act on that knowledge by applying coping strategies through which they can regulate their responses to the advertisement and their food choice behavior. Educational intervention programs should therefore not only increase their advertising knowledge, but also provide them with the *ability* and *motivation* to effectively engage their advertising coping strategies and successfully resist advertising for highly appealing but unhealthy foods.

Explaining and predicting children's food advertising coping strategies

Figure 5.1 depicts how advertising knowledge, ability (i.e., emotion control and perceived competence), and motivation to use advertising coping strategies are expected to interact in explaining and predicting children's actual use of coping strategies when confronted with food advertising (see Rozendaal, 2016). Below I will elaborate more on the importance of ability and motivation as predictors of children's actual use of food advertising coping strategies. Also, I will discuss a set of theory-based intervention techniques (i.e., emotion labeling, implementation intentions, and self-persuasion) that are expected to be effective in stimulating children's ability and motivation to use advertising coping strategies, and which could be translated into practical educational materials in order to make children more aware of the effects of food advertising.

Ability to apply advertising coping strategies

Insights from developmental theories suggest that children's ability to enact coping strategies depends largely on their cognitive skills (Moses & Baldwin, 2005; Rozendaal et al., 2011). To enact coping strategies, children need to have the cognitive control to stop their initial emotional responses to the advertising message and instead react alternatively (i.e., enact coping strategies). In the literature, this process is also called the "stop-and-think reaction" (Rozendaal et al., 2011), because it requires that children control their emotional reactions ("stop") and then come up with a strategy to cope with the situation ("think"). The upper half of Figure 5.1 depicts the two mechanisms that are assumed by the model to play

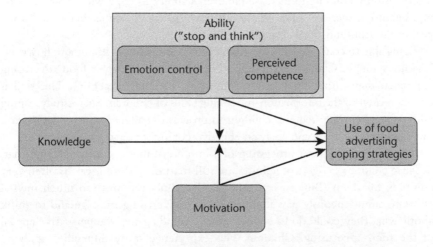

FIGURE 5.1 Predictors of children's use of (food) advertising coping strategies.

a key role in children's ability to "stop and think" while confronted with food advertising: *emotion control* and *competence*.

The "stop" part of the stop-and-think reaction is closely related to the emotion regulation skills of children (Rozendaal et al., 2011). Emotion regulation is the ability to cope with and express both positive and negative emotions. This skill only reaches an adult level in the last phase of adolescence (Diamond, 2002). Emotion regulation is expected to play an important role in children's ability to stop and think about food advertisements, particularly because so much of the content in contemporary food advertisements is centered on emotional cues (see Chapters 1 and 2). Moreover, the evolutionary preference for the often-advertised foods high in salt, sugar, and fat entails a strong pre-programmed impulsive psychological affective reaction, which further emphasizes the relevance of emotion regulation in children's ability to resist its appeal (Folkvord, 2016). Children who are less able to control their emotions will easily be overwhelmed by the emotional aspects of food advertising and therefore less able to control their coping behavior. It is therefore assumed that the ability to control advertising-induced emotions is an important predictor of children's actual use of coping strategies when confronted with food advertising.

Although emotion regulation skills naturally develop when children mature, research showed that these skills are trainable and can be improved at any age (e.g., Greenberg, Kusche, Cook, & Quamma, 1995; Izard et al., 2008). Social-emotional development programs (e.g., PATHS, Head Start, and mindfulness) offer useful techniques in this respect. In these programs, children learn to become aware of and express their emotions. The premise behind this is that increasing children's ability to understand and label their feeling states or emotion experiences will increase their conscious control of them (Greenberg et al., 1995; Izard et al., 2008). Thus, the labeling of emotions may be an effective intervention technique to increase children's ability to cope with food advertising, because it increases their emotion regulation which can facilitate the "stop" part of the stop-and-think response.

Being able to control advertising-induced emotions is thus important; however, it is not enough. Children should also be able to activate their food advertising coping strategies (the "think" part of the stop-and-think reaction). This skill is closely related to the information-processing skills of children. Successfully coping with food advertising requires children to process the advertising message and, at the same time, activate and apply an effective coping strategy.

Theories of children's processing of commercial media content suggest that, because children's cognitive abilities are still maturing, this process is often very complex for them (Buijzen et al., 2010). It simply requires too much mental effort to simultaneously pay attention to the advertising message and to think about what they could do to cope with or defend against the persuasive appeal of the food advertising. Children who experience more difficulties applying coping strategies are likely to feel less competent in regulating their behavior. In other words, if children don't know which strategies they can use to deal with food advertising, then they probably also feel less capable of regulating their own behavioral responses to food advertising. Insights from theories on behavior regulation and behavior change suggest that, when someone's perceived competence to perform a behavior is low, he or she is less likely to actually perform that behavior (Ajzen, 1991; Bandura, 1997; Baumeister & Vohs, 2007; Deci & Ryan, 2000; Ryan & Deci, 2000). In line with these theories, it is therefore assumed that perceived competence to effectively enact coping strategies is an important predictor of children's actual use of coping strategies when confronted with food advertising.

A technique that could increase children's ability to actually enact their food advertising coping strategies, even if the deployable mental capacity is low, as is the case with children, is implementation intentions. Implementation intentions are simple if–then plans that specify when and how one's goal will be put into practice (i.e., "If situation X occurs, then I will respond in this way"; Gollwitzer, 1999). With practice, this process can become a mental routine and subsequently lead to behavior change in relatively automatic ways, while using few cognitive resources. The efficacy of this behavior change technique has been demonstrated convincingly in various domains (e.g., Gollwitzer & Sheeran, 2006; Hagger & Luszczynska, 2014), yet has only recently been related to the goal of coping with advertising (Hudders et al., 2016).

Implementation intentions may be a powerful intervention technique to increase children's ability to cope with food advertising, as it can help them to actually enact a coping strategy (the "think" part of stop and think) by relying on simple and low-demanding if–then heuristics.

Motivation to apply advertising coping strategies

Theories on behavior regulation and behavior change suggest that, without motivation or intention to do so, people are unlikely to put effort in regulating their behavior (Ajzen, 1991; Baumeister & Vohs, 2007; Deci & Ryan, 2000; Ryan & Deci, 2000). Thus, children who are less motivated to apply coping strategies while confronted with food advertising are less likely to regulate and adjust their responses in order to be more skeptical and avoidant towards food advertising. In line with behavior regulation and behavior change theories (Ajzen, 1991; Baumeister & Vohs, 2007; Deci & Ryan, 2000; Ryan & Deci, 2000), it is therefore assumed that children's motivation to apply coping strategies is an important predictor of children's actual use of (food) advertising coping strategies.

A common technique used in persuasion research to motivate people to change their behavior is by providing arguments why it is important to change (Petty & Wegener, 1991). However, when faced with counter-attitudinal arguments, most people will not comply (Aronson, 1999). Therefore, it is expected that providing children with arguments why it is important to critically cope with advertising (to which they generally hold positive attitudes; e.g., Rozendaal et al., 2013) will actually not motivate them to activate coping strategies.

Self-persuasion may overcome this problem (Aronson, 1999). Self-persuasion stems from Festinger's cognitive dissonance theory (Festinger, 1957), which states that dissonance (an unpleasant feeling) is aroused when individuals notice inconsistency between their attitudes and their behavior. To reduce dissonance, people try to restore balance by changing their attitudes or behavior. Self-persuasion uses this principle by asking people to argue in favor of a desired behavior ("Write down two arguments that stress why it's important to be critical about advertising"). Once a relevant situation occurs (when confronted with advertising), people have the tendency to rely on these self-generated arguments in order to avoid dissonance.

Self-persuasion is a powerful technique because it increases people's intrinsic motivation to change their behavior or attitudes (Mussweiler & Neumann, 2000). It has been shown to be effective in a wide variety of contexts (e.g., condom use, smoking behavior, alcohol use; Banerjee & Greene, 2007; Briñol, McCaslin, & Petty, 2012; Müller et al., 2009; Stone, Aronson, Crain, Winslow, & Fried, 1994), yet has not been applied in the context of food advertising or with children. Children as young as 4 can already experience dissonance (Egan, Santos, & Bloom, 2007). Therefore, self-persuasion may be an effective intervention technique to increase children's motivation to enact food advertising coping strategies.

Empowering children to cope with food advertising through advertising disclosures

Another way to increase children's advertising defenses, in particular with regard to embedded types of (digital) food advertising (i.e., advergames, brand placement), is to give a sponsorship or advertising disclosure alongside the advertising message. A disclosure can take various forms, such as an advertising break on television or a disclaimer identifying the presence of commercial content on a website or in a game (An & Stern, 2011). Sponsorship disclosures are assumed to empower consumers, both adults and children, because they may activate their awareness and knowledge of the commercial nature of sponsored media content (An & Stern, 2011; Campbell & Evans, 2018). Specifically, the warning can facilitate recognition of the commercial message and trigger children to think about the purpose of the sponsored media content. When they realize that this is to persuade, children may adopt a more critical attitude, which helps them to make more deliberate and autonomous decisions.

Only a few studies have investigated the effectiveness of sponsorship disclosures in activating children's persuasion knowledge for food advertising (An & Stern, 2011; De Pauw, Hudders, & Cauberghe, 2018; Panic et al., 2013; Van Reijmersdal, Boerman, Buijzen, & Rozendaal, 2017; Vanwesenbeeck, Opree, & Smits, 2017). The findings of these studies do not provide conclusive evidence. While some studies did find a disclosure to be effective in increasing children's understanding of or resistance toward food-related sponsored content, others did not find such an effect (An & Stern, 2011; De Pauw et al., 2018; Folkvord et al., 2017; Panic et al., 2013;

Van Reijmersdal et al., 2017; Van Reijmersdal, Rozendaal, Hudders, Cauberghe, & Van Berlo, 2018; Vanwesenbeeck, Walrave, & Ponnet, 2017).

A pioneering study by An and Stern (2011) on the effectiveness of advertising forewarnings among children has shown that the presence of a warning in a food advergame ("Advertisement: the game and other activities on this website contain message about the products sold by Kraft") made children more resistant to its effects; more specifically, the children who played an advergame in which the warning was present showed less desire for the advertised Honey-Comb cereals. It is important to note that the warning did not cause the children to understand the persuasive intent of the game better, but primes them with the message that the game is an advertising. This indicates that a sponsorship disclosure in an advergame makes children less susceptible to the game itself, without them being aware of the commercial nature. This finding is interesting. It demonstrates that resistance to advertising does not need to be a conscious process, but that children can also resist the influence of advertising at a subconscious level.

More recently, Van Reijmersdal et al. (2018) investigated the effects of sponsorship disclosures for a relatively new phenomenon: social media influencer marketing. Social media influencers (e.g., beauty bloggers, video game vloggers, unboxers, instafamous) who mention, use, or promote unhealthy food products in their videos or posts, are an important topic of concerns regarding fairness (Federal Trade Commission, 2013). These influencers have millions of young viewers and many influencers are used by brands, in particular unhealthy food brands, to advertise their products (Folkvord, Bevelander, Rozendaal, & Hermans, in press; McAlone, 2017).

In their study, Van Reijmersdal and colleagues (2018) investigated the effects of sponsorship disclosures on children's (10–13 years) ability to understand that social media influencer videos on YouTube are sponsored. They also investigated how sponsorship disclosures affect children's attitudes toward the sponsoring brand, the video, and the influencer. Van Reijmersdal et al. specifically focused on social influencer videos, including sponsored content for unhealthy food brands: the soft drink brand Fanta, and the fish stick brand Iglo. In the Fanta video, a male YouTuber goes to a theme park to do a challenge for Fanta. He makes a graffiti of the Fanta logo and designs a new logo for Fanta while riding a rollercoaster. In the Iglo video, a group of three male YouTubers are challenged to create the largest fish stick sponsored by Iglo. To get inspiration, they first buy a lot of Iglo fish sticks in the supermarket. They bring these to a brainstorm session in which they determine their strategy. Then they go to a restaurant to prepare the largest fish stick of the world.

Prior to or concurrent with the start of the video, the children were shown the following sponsorship disclosure "X [name of influencer] is paid by brand Y to advertise their products in his video." The disclosure was visible for 10 seconds at the top of the screen. In the disclosure prior to the start condition, the disclosure was visible only before the videos started in a white font on a black background also for 10 seconds. Concurrent with the start of the video conditions, the disclosure appeared after the start of videos at the same position on the screen, in the same size, also in white font, and also for 10 seconds, in a black box.

Van Reijmersdal et al. (2018) were interested in the effectiveness of sponsorship disclosures with different timings (i.e., disclosure displayed prior to the start of sponsored videos or concurrent with the start of the videos), because the timing of a disclosure is assumed to be an important determinant of disclosure noticeability and thus of a child's opportunity to process the disclosure and the extent to which the disclosure triggers advertising literacy (Boerman, Van Reijmersdal, & Neijens, 2014; Choi, Bang, Wojdynski, Lee, & Keib, 2018; De Pauw et al., 2018; MacInnis, Moorman, & Jaworski, 1991). They expected that, compared to a disclosure concurrent with the start of the video, a disclosure prior to the start of the video is more easy to process for children and as a result more effective. After all, when the content of the video has not started yet, children also cannot be distracted by that content, which increases the likelihood that they pay attention to the disclosure.

Results showed that a disclosure that is shown prior to the start of the videos indeed leads to more visual attention than a disclosure that is shown concurrent with the start of the videos. Consequently, the disclosure prior to the start of the videos is better processed, as indicated by disclosure memory, which then leads to a better understanding that the content is sponsored. This understanding evokes a more critical attitude toward the sponsored content in the video, and finally results in less positive attitudes toward the unhealthy food brands, the videos, and the influencers.

The study by Van Reijmersdal et al. (2018) shows that timing of the disclosure (i.e., before or concurrent with the start of a sponsored video) is an important factor for disclosure effectiveness. However, many questions with regard to the design (e.g., visual/auditory, color, message) of effective advertising disclosures have been left unanswered. For example, how should a disclosure be formulated in order to be understandable for children? In order to be effective, it is all the more important to make sure that children understand the meaning of sponsorship disclosures. Research has revealed that if children don't understand its meaning, a disclosure will not be successful in terms of stimulating advertising recognition and (certainly not) in terms of critical reflection (De Jans et al., 2018).

Conclusion

The current chapter shed light on the role of advertising literacy in their susceptibility to food advertising. It emphasized the need to empower children to defend against highly appealing but unhealthy food advertising through advertising literacy education. It also showed that, in order to help children defend against food advertising, educational intervention programs should not only increase children's advertising knowledge but also provide them with the ability and motivation to effectively engage their food advertising coping strategies. Finally, the chapter discussed the implementation of advertising disclosures that improve recognition of embedded types of food advertising (e.g., food advergames, food product place-ments in influencer videos) and help children activate their critical processing mechanisms.

References

Ajzen, I. (1991). The theory of planned behavior. *Organizational Behavior and Human Decision Processes, 50*(2), 179–211.

An, S., & Stern, S. (2011). Mitigating the effects of advergames on children. *Journal of Advertising, 40*(1), 43–56.

Aronson, E. (1999). The power of self-persuasion. *American Psychologist, 54*(11), 875–884.

Auty, S., & Lewis, C. (2004). Exploring children's choice: The reminder effect of product placement. *Psychology & Marketing, 21*(9), 697–713.

Bandura, A. (1997). *Self-efficacy: The exercise of control.* New York, NY: W. H. Freeman/ Times Books/Henry Holt.

Banerjee, S. C., & Greene, K. (2007). Anti-smoking initiatives: Effects of analysis versus production media literacy interventions on smoking-related attitude, norm, and behav-ioral intention. *Health Communication, 22*, 37–48.

Baumeister, R. F., & Vohs, K. D. (2007). Self-regulation, ego depletion, and motivation. *Social and Personality Psychology Compass, 1*(1), 115–128.

Boerman, S. C., Van Reijmersdal, E. A., & Neijens, P. C. (2014). Effects of sponsorship disclosure timing on the processing of sponsored content: A study on the effectiveness of European disclosure regulations. *Psychology & Marketing, 31*(3), 214–224.

Boyland, E. J., & Whalen, R. (2015). Food advertising to children and its effects on diet: Review of recent prevalence and impact data. *Pediatric Diabetes, 16*(5), 331–337.

Briñol, P., McCaslin, M. J., & Petty, R. E. (2012). Self-generated persuasion: Effects of the target and direction of arguments. *Journal of Personality and Social Psychology, 102*, 925–940.

Brucks, M., Armstrong, G. M., & Goldberg, M. E. (1988). Children's use of cognitive defenses against television advertising: A cognitive response approach. *Journal of Consumer Research, 14*, 471–482.

Buijzen, M., & Valkenburg, P. M. (2003). The effects of television advertising on mate-rialism, parent–child conflict, and unhappiness: A review of research. *Journal of Applied Developmental Psychology, 24*(4), 437–456.

Buijzen, M., Van Reijmersdal, E. A., & Owen, L. H. (2010). Introducing the PCMC model: An investigative framework for young people's processing of commercial media content. *Communication Theory, 20*, 427–450.

Calvert, S. L. (2008). Children as consumers: Advertising and marketing. *The Future of Children, 18*(1), 205–234.

Campbell, C., & Evans, N. J. (2018). The role of a companion banner and sponsorship transparency in recognizing and evaluating article-style native advertising. *Journal of Interactive Marketing, 43*, 17–32.

Choi, D., Bang, H., Wojdynski, B. W., Lee, Y., & Keib, K. M. (2018). How brand dis-closure timing and brand prominence influence consumer's intention to share branded entertainment content. *Journal of Interactive Marketing, 42*, 18–31.

D'Alessio, M., Laghi, F., & Baiocco, R. (2009). Attitudes toward TV advertising: A meas-ure for children. *Journal of Applied Developmental Psychology, 30*(4), 409–418.

Deci, E. L., & Ryan, R. M. (2000). The" what" and" why" of goal pursuits: Human needs and the self-determination of behavior. *Psychological Inquiry, 11*(4), 227–268.

De Jans, S., Hudders, L., & Cauberghe, V. (2017). Advertising literacy training: The immediate versus delayed effects on children's responses to product placement. *European Journal of Marketing*, *51*(11/12), 2156–2174.

De Jans, S., Van de Sompel, D., Hudders, L., & Cauberghe, V. (2017). Advertising targeting young children: An overview of 10 years of research (2006–2016). *International Journal of Advertising*, 1–34.

De Jans, S., Vanwesenbeeck, I., Cauberghe, V., Hudders, L., Rozendaal, E., & van Reijmersdal, E. A. (2018). The development and testing of a child-inspired advertising disclosure to alert children to digital and embedded advertising. *Journal of Advertising*, 1–15.

De Pauw, P., Hudders, L., & Cauberghe, V. (2018). Disclosing brand placement to young children. *International Journal of Advertising*, *37*(4), 508–525.

Diamond, A. (2002). Normal development of prefrontal cortex from birth to young adulthood: Cognitive functions, anatomy, and biochemistry. In D.T. Stuss & R.T. Knight (Eds.), *Principles of frontal lobe function* (pp. 466–503). New York, NY: Oxford University Press.

Egan, L. C., Santos, L. R., & Bloom, P. (2007) The origins of cognitive dissonance: Evidence from children and monkeys. *Psychological Science*, *18*(11), 978–983.

Federal Trade Commission. (2013). *.Com disclosures. How to make effective disclosure in digital advertising*. Retrieved from http://www.ftc.gov/sites/default/files/attachments/press-releases/ftc-staff-revises-onlineadvertising-disclosure-guidelines/130312dotcomdisclosures.pdf

Festinger, L. (1957). *A theory of cognitive dissonance*. Stanford, CA: Stanford University Press.

Folkvord, F. (2016). *Children's reactivity to embedded food cues in advergames* (unpublished doctoral dissertation). Radboud University, The Netherlands.

Folkvord, F., Bevelander, K. E., Rozendaal, E., & Hermans, R. (2019, forthcoming). Children's bonding with popular YouTube vloggers and their attitudes towards brand and product endorsements in vlogs: An explorative study. *Young Consumers*.

Folkvord, F., Lupiáñez-Villanueva, F., Codagnone, C., Bogliacino, F., Veltri, G., & Gaskell, G. (2017). Does a 'protective'message reduce the impact of an advergame promoting unhealthy foods to children? An experimental study in Spain and The Netherlands. *Appetite*, *112*, 117–123.

Friestad, M., & Wright, P. (1994). The persuasion knowledge model: How people cope with persuasion attempts. *Journal of Consumer Research*, 1–31.

Gollwitzer, P. M. (1999). Implementation intentions: Strong effects of simple plans. *American Psychologist*, *54*(7), 493.

Gollwitzer, P. M., & Sheeran, P. (2006). Implementation intentions and goal achievement: A meta-analysis of effects and processes. *Advances in Experimental Social Psychology*, *38*, 69–119.

Greenberg, M. T., Kusche, C. A., Cook, E. T., & Quamma, J. P. (1995). Promoting emotional competence in school-aged children: The effects of the PATHS curriculum. *Development and Psychopathology*, *7*, 117–136.

Hagger, M. S., & Luszczynska, A. (2014). Implementation intention and action planning interventions in health contexts: State of the research and proposals for the way forward. *Applied Psychology: Health and Well-Being*, *6*(1), 1–47.

Harris, J. L., Brownell, K. D., & Bargh, J. A. (2009). The food marketing defense model: Integrating psychological research to protect youth and inform public policy. *Social Issues and Policy Review*, *3*(1), 211–271.

Hudders, L., Cauberghe, V., & Panic, K. (2016). How advertising literacy training affect children's responses to television commercials versus advergames. *International Journal of Advertising*, 1–23.

Hudders, L., De Pauw, P., Cauberghe, V., Panic, K., Zarouali, B., & Rozendaal, E. (2017). Shedding new light on how advertising literacy can affect children's processing of embedded advertising formats: A future research agenda. *Journal of Advertising*, *46*(2), 333–349.

Izard, C. E., King, K. A., Trentacosta, C. J., Morgan, J. K., Laurenceau, J. P., Krauthamer-Ewing, E. S., & Finlon, K. J. (2008). Accelerating the development of emotion competence in Head Start children: Effects on adaptive and maladaptive behavior. *Development and Psychopathology*, *20*(01), 369–397.

Jeong, S. H., Cho, H., & Hwang, Y. (2012). Media literacy interventions: A meta-analytic review. *Journal of Communication*, *62*(3), 454–472.

John, D. R. (1999). Consumer socialization of children: A retrospective look at twenty-five years of research. *Journal of Consumer Research*, *26*, 183–213.

Kunkel, D., Wilcox, B. L., Cantor, J., Palmer, E., Linn, S., & Dowrick, P. (2004). *Report of the APA Task Force on advertising and children*. Washington, DC: American Psychological Association.

Lang, A. (2000). The limited capacity model of mediated message processing. *Journal of communication*, *50*(1), 46–70.

Livingstone, S., & Helsper, E.J. (2006). Does advertising literacy mediate the effects of advertising on children? A critical examination of two linked research literatures in relation to obesity and food choice. *Journal of Communication*, *56*, 560–584.

MacInnis, D. J., Moorman, C., & Jaworski, B. J. (1991). Enhancing and measuring consumers' motivation, opportunity, and ability to process brand information from ads. *The Journal of Marketing*, 32–53.

Mallinckrodt, V., & Mizerski, D. (2007). The effects of playing an advergame on young children's perceptions, preferences, and requests. *Journal of Advertising*, *36*(2), 87–100.

McAlone, N. (2017). These are the 18 most popular YouTube stars in the world — and some are making millions. *Business Insider*. Retrieved from https://www.businessinsider.nl/most-popular-youtuber-stars-salaries-2017/?international=true&r=US

Mizerski, D., Wang, S., Lee, A., & Lambert, C. (2017). Young children as consumers: Their vulnerability to persuasion and its effect on their choices. In: C. V. Jansson-Boyd, & M. J. Zawisza (Eds.). *Routledge international handbook of consumer psychology* (pp. 327–346). New York, NY: Routledge.

Moore, E. S. (2004). Children and the changing world of advertising. *Journal of business Ethics*, *52*(2), 161–167.

Moses, L. J., & Baldwin, D. A. (2005). What can the study of cognitive development reveal about children's ability to appreciate and cope with advertising? *Journal of Public Policy & Marketing*, *24*, 186–201.

Müller, B. C. N., van Baaren, R. B., Ritter, S. M., Woud, M. L., Bergmann, H., Harakeh, Z., Engels, R. C. M. E., & Dijksterhuis, A. (2009). Tell me why. . . The influence of self-involvement on short term smoking behaviour. *Addictive Behaviors*, *34*, 427–431.

Mussweiler, T., & Neumann, R. (2000). Sources of mental contamination: Comparing the effects of self-generated versus externally provided primes. *Journal of Experimental Social Psychology*, *36*, 194–206.

Nairn, A., & Fine, C. (2008) Who's messing with my mind? The implications of dual-process models for ethics of advertising to children. *International Journal of Advertising*, *27*, 447–470.

Nelson, M. R. (2016). Developing persuasion knowledge by teaching advertising literacy in primary school. *Journal of Advertising, 45*(2), 169–182.

Owen, L., Lewis, C., Auty, S., & Buijzen, M. (2013). Is children's understanding of nontraditional advertising comparable to their understanding of television advertising?. *Journal of Public Policy & Marketing, 32*(2), 195–206.

Panic, K., Cauberghe, V., & De Pelsmacker, P. (2013). Comparing TV ads and advergames targeting children: The impact of persuasion knowledge on behavioral responses. *Journal of Advertising, 42*(2–3), 264–273.

Petty, R. E., & Wegener, D. T. (1991). Thought systems, argument quality, and persuasion. In: R. S. Wyer & T. K. Srull (Eds.), *Advances in social cognition* (pp. 147–161). New York: Psychology Press.

Roberts, M., & Pettigrew, S. (2013). Psychosocial influences on children's food consumption. *Psychology & Marketing, 30*(2), 103–120.

Rozendaal, E. (2016, June). *The development of a school-based intervention to empower children to cope with advertising.* Paper presented at the annual conference of the International Communication Association, Fukuoka, Japan.

Rozendaal, E., Buijzen, M., & Valkenburg, P.M. (2012). Think-aloud method superior to thought-listing in increasing children's advertising defenses. *Human Communication Research, 38,* 198–220.

Rozendaal, E., Lapierre, M. A., Van Reijmersdal, E. A., & Buijzen, M. (2011). Reconsidering advertising literacy as a defense against advertising effects. *Media Psychology, 14,* 333–354.

Rozendaal, E., Slot, N., van Reijmersdal, E. A., & Buijzen, M. (2013). Children's responses to advertising in social games. *Journal of Advertising, 42*(2–3), 142–154.

Ryan, R. M., & Deci, E. L. (2000). Self-determination theory and the facilitation of intrinsic motivation, social development, and well-being. *American Psychologist, 55*(1), 68.

Stone, J., Aronson, E., Crain, A. L., Winslow, M. P., & Fried, C. B. (1994). Inducing hypocrisy as a means of encouraging young adults to use condoms. *Personality and Social Psychology Bulletin, 20*(1), 116–128.

Valkenburg, P. M., & Buijzen, M. (2005). Identifying determinants of young children's brand awareness: Television, parents, and peers. *Journal of Applied Developmental Psychology, 26*(4), 456–468.

Van Reijmersdal, E. A., Boerman, S. C., Buijzen, M., & Rozendaal, E. (2017). This is advertising! Effects of disclosing television brand placement on adolescents. *Journal of Youth and Adolescence, 46*(2), 328–342.

Van Reijmersdal, E. A., Rozendaal, E., & Buijzen, M. (2012). Effects of prominence, involvement, and persuasion knowledge on children's cognitive and affective responses to advergames. *Journal of Interactive Marketing, 26* (1), 33–42.

Van Reijmersdal, E. A., Rozendaal, E., Hudders, L., Cauberghe, V., & Van Berlo, Z. M. C. (2018, March). This video is sponsored! An eye tracking study on the effects of disclosure timing on children's persuasion knowledge. *Manuscript presented at the American Academy of Advertising annual conference in New York*, USA.

Vanwesenbeeck, I., Opree, S. J., & Smits, T. (2017). Can disclosures aid children's recognition of TV and website advertising? In: V. Zabkar & M. Eisend (Eds.), *Advances in advertising research VIII* (pp. 45–57). Wiesbaden: Gabler.

Vanwesenbeeck, I., Walrave, M., & Ponnet, K. (2017). Children and advergames: The role of product involvement, prior brand attitude, persuasion knowledge and game attitude in purchase intentions and changing attitudes. *International Journal of Advertising, 36*(4), 520–541.

Verhellen, Y., Oates, C., De Pelsmacker, P., & Dens, N. (2014). Children's responses to traditional versus hybrid advertising formats: The moderating role of persuasion knowledge. *Journal of Consumer Policy*, *37*(2), 235–255.

Waiguny, M. K., Nelson, M. R., & Terlutter, R. (2012). Entertainment matters! The relationship between challenge and persuasiveness of an advergame for children. *Journal of Marketing Communications*, *18*(1), 69–89.

Waiguny, M. K., & Terlutter, R. (2011). Differences in children's processing of advergames and TV commercials. In: S. Okazaki (Ed.), *Advances in advertising research (vol. 2)* (pp. 35–51). Wiesbaden: Gabler.

Wollslager, M. E. (2009). Children's awareness of online advertising on Neopets: The effect of media literacy training on recall. *Studies in Media & Information Literacy Education*, *9*(2), 31–53.

Wright, P., Friestad, M., & Boush, D. M. (2005). The development of marketplace persuasion knowledge in children, adolescents, and young adults. *Journal of Public Policy & Marketing*, *24*, 222–233.

6

EMPOWERING CONSUMERS TO CHOOSE WHAT THEY WANT

Toward behavior change in a food advertising environment

Dr. Harm Veling and Dr. Natalia Lawrence

Many people have a desire to change their everyday dietary choices. People may want to reduce their intake of foods high in fat, sugar, or salt (HFSS food) to lose weight (Santos, Sniehotta, Marques, Carraça, & Teixeira, 2017), or reduce consumption of meat products for health, environmental, or moral reasons (e.g., Rozin, Markwith, & Stoess, 1997). At the same time, these products are widely and effectively advertised and promoted, which is associated with demand for these products and consumption (e.g., Andreyeva, Kelly, & Harris, 2011; Brester & Schroeder, 1995). This raises the question of whether and how people can inhibit their responses to these kinds of products in an environment where these food advertisements are omnipresent. Indeed, maintaining changes in dietary choices across longer periods of time may be very difficult (e.g., Elfhag & Rössner, 2005). For instance, despite continuous efforts to develop effective behavior change weight loss interventions, interventions to date that aim to establish changes across time, still require much improvement (e.g., Wilfley, Hayes, Balantekin, Van Buren, & Epstein, 2018).

There may be many reasons for the difficulty with changing dietary choices, but it seems very likely that this difficulty is partly caused because choices for food, and food consumption more generally, are shaped by basic learning mechanisms that create preferences for HFSS foods and branded meat products (e.g., hamburgers from Burger King), because these foods contain intrinsically rewarding properties such as sugar, salt, and fat (e.g., Epstein, Carr, Lin, & Fletcher, 2011). In addition, many of these kinds of products are often heavily advertised and promoted (Story & French, 2004), and exposure to such foods can be difficult to avoid, so that these learned reward associations can steer behavior across many contexts. Moreover, exposure to a brand name of a heavily advertised product can increase perceived taste for this product (e.g., Robinson, Borzekowski, Matheson, & Kraemer, 2007). Thus, from this perspective, advertising and food promotion pose difficulties for people to inhibit their responses to HFSS foods by exposing them persistently to these rewarding products, and by increasing taste preferences for them.

In the present chapter, we will first describe learning mechanisms that shape food preferences that contribute to the difficulty for many people to modify their consumption behavior. Then, we will discuss two qualitatively different behavior change approaches to modify people's food consumption, called *nudging* (Thaler & Sunstein, 2008) and *boosting* (Hertwig & Grüne-Yanoff, 2017). Next, we will discuss in more detail one intervention, go/no-go (GNG) training (Veling, Lawrence, Chen, Van Koningsbruggen, & Holland, 2017), which seems successful in modifying food consumption by targeting the learnt affective and behavioral responses that contribute to people's difficulty in changing their dietary choices. We will discuss the basic research findings of this training, and present a first impression of how this training may be used as a boost to change food consumption among large groups of consumers who want to change their food preferences. We will primarily focus on how to reduce preferences for HFSS foods low in nutrients, as these foods are heavily advertised despite the fact that they are broadly considered unhealthy (e.g., Story & French, 2004).

Basic learning mechanisms shaping food consumption

Two basic learning mechanisms that greatly contribute to the development of food preferences and food-related changes in motivation are pavlovian and instrumental (or operant) conditioning (Berridge & Robinson, 2003; Rangel, 2013). HFSS foods such as a candy bar contain ingredients such as sugar and fat that are intrinsically rewarding, i.e., they stimulate opioid and dopamine transmission in the brain's reward circuits and elicit feelings of pleasure ("liking") in the consumer (Berridge, 2009). Two important things happen as a result of this rewarding experience: First, sensory cues (e.g., sights, smells) present at the same time as the food become associated with its rewarding effects. Food packaging and brands are examples of visual cues that frequently accompany HFSS food intake. These cues may hence trigger responses associated with the food, such as salivation, physiological arousal, and food craving (pavlovian conditioning). The conditioned responses to food cues can occur unconsciously or consciously, are robust, and can develop after as little as one conditioning session (Van Gucht, Vansteenwegen, Van den Bergh, & Beckers, 2008).

The food-associated cues can also acquire rewarding and motivational properties themselves ("incentive salience"), such that some individuals' attention is grabbed by the cues and they become "energized" and more willing to work for the cue and its reward (Berridge, 2009). People differ in their reactivity to food-associated cues (e.g., how much they salivate, experience cravings, show increased brain activity in dopamine-rich reward circuits) and substantial evidence suggests that those who show greater "food cue reactivity" eat more and gain more weight (Boswell & Kober, 2016).

The second important consequence of consuming a rewarding HFSS food is that choices for these foods can be reinforced via so-called instrumental conditioning. This means that the act (motor response) of choosing this food in some way, e.g., picking up and buying a candy bar, is reinforced by linking this act to an eventually rewarding outcome such as the taste and pleasure resulting from sugar consumption and the rewarding postingestional feeling of satiety (e.g., Berridge, 2009; Epstein et al., 2011; Rozin & Zellner, 1985). The food-directed motor response is said to be "positively reinforced" and is more likely to be performed again in the future. This instrumental learning works alongside the pavlovian conditioned responses described above, and together they may quickly lead to the creation of pavlovian biases where the reward-predicting stimulus, for instance, the visual presentation of a branded food item in a shop, grabs one's attention, elicits physiological and motor arousal, and more or less automatically stimulates responses toward obtaining the food (e.g., Watson, Wiers, Hommel, & De Wit, 2014). Cues associated with a food reward can increase activity in the brain's motor cortex very quickly, triggering approach responses that can be very difficult to inhibit (Freeman, Razhas, & Aron, 2014).

Watson and colleagues (2014, p. 140) describe how these learning mechanisms may contribute to food marketing effects: "*seeing the golden arches of the McDonald's restaurant chain on a billboard may remind one of cheeseburgers, the thought of which triggers the action of going to McDonald's, even when one is already fully sated.*" Note that these processes may happen without much deliberation. Once strong stimulus–response links have been acquired, such as between the visual perception of a food item/its associated brand and selection of the food item, or between cues signaling the presence of food, and positive affective reactions toward the food, these associations may guide behavior irrespective of people's goals or intentions to choose the food (e.g., Friese, Wänke, & Plessner, 2006; Strack & Deutsch, 2004; Sullivan, Hutcherson, Harris, & Rangel, 2015). Thus, due to the rapid and automatic nature of this learnt behavioral response to food cues, it can become very hard to change eating behavior (e.g., reduce candy bar intake) even when this change is strongly desired by an individual (e.g., Stroebe, Van Koningsbruggen, Papies, & Aarts, 2013).

Pavlovian food advertisements

The basic learning mechanisms outlined above may explain at least two observations about our current food environment. First, it may explain why foods high in energy density, as well as cues for these kinds of foods such as brand names and advertisements, are so widely visibly presented. Pavlovian biases for these kinds of rewarding foods or food cues are quickly acquired and can strongly stimulate consumption (Van den Akker, Schyns, & Jansen, 2018). When foods have fewer intrinsically rewarding ingredients, as may be the case for lower-calorie (but more nutritious) foods such as vegetables, pavlovian biases may develop less strongly (Watson, Wiers, Hommel, Gerdes, & De Wit, 2017). Thus, from a commercial perspective it seems very worthwhile and effective to particularly offer and promote high-calorie foods very visibly instead of less rewarding foods, so that learned associations can steer behavior. It may also explain why many people, who are surrounded by these food-associated cues, find it so difficult to regulate their food intake. Pavlovian biases should work relatively automatically and independently of people's goals to eat healthily, and may stimulate consumption irrespective of such goals. These observations raise the question of whether and how it would be possible to establish long-term changes in people's food consumption away from the heavily advertised high-calorie foods (e.g., Story & French, 2004), towards more healthful lower-calorie foods.

Nudging behavior change

To address the question of how to best change food consumption of large groups of people, two qualitatively different approaches can be distinguished. The first approach is to implement changes in the environment where people make food choices (i.e., in the choice architecture) that facilitate consumption of some kinds of foods (e.g., low-calorie foods) over other kinds of food (e.g., high-calorie foods). One version of this approach has become very popular under the label *nudging* (Thaler & Sunstein, 2008). Nudging means that the choice architecture is changed in such a manner that some choices are made easier than other choices, while at the same time options are not removed (or forbidden) so that people's freedom of choice is not impaired (for an alternative conceptualization of the environmental approach, see Hollands et al., 2017). Moreover, nudging emphasizes behavior change without using financial incentives (for an alternative approach focusing on taxes, see Brownell et al., 2009). A typical example would be to place healthful products more visibly in a shop (e.g., at eye level in a grocery store) at the expense of products considered unhealthy, to boost their consumption (e.g., Wilson, Buckley, Buckley, & Bogomolova, 2016). In essence this means using the marketing strategies traditionally applied to HFSS foods to more nutritious healthy foods. Several studies suggest that this approach can be effective in stimulating choices for relatively healthy foods (e.g., Thorndike, Riis, Sonnenberg, & Levy, 2014). Another environmental intervention, focusing on consumption volume rather than on choice, is to provide people with smaller plates or packaged portions so that they might eat less food (e.g., Holden, Zlatevska, & Dubelaar, 2016).

Apart from such environmental interventions, it is also possible to provide people with short informational messages in the choice architecture, e.g., at the point of purchase, to steer their behavior (e.g., Carter, Bignardi, Hollands, & Marteau, 2018). For instance, research has shown that a short informational message on a menu card in a restaurant indicating which dishes contain relatively few calories stimulates choices for such dishes among people who have the goal to lose weight (Papies & Veling, 2013; see also Papies & Hamstra, 2010). These messages are not always effective (Dorresteijn, Van der Graaf, Zheng, Spiering, &

Visseren, 2013), but seem effective when they activate goals, such as losing weight, which people endorse (Papies & Veling, 2013). This finding suggests an important asymmetry between promoting HFSS foods versus lower-calorie foods: Promotion of HFSS foods by emphasizing their tasty nature may stimulate consumption even among consumers who intend to limit their intake of these kinds of foods (e.g., Stroebe et al., 2013), whereas promotion of lower-calorie foods may only work to stimulate consumption among those consumers who are already motivated to reduce their calorie intake (Papies & Veling, 2013). Finally, a recent meta-analysis of healthy-eating nudges suggests that behavioral strategies (e.g., changing the portion size or the convenience of foods) are more effective than cognitive nudges (e.g., making foods more visible or changing how they are labeled; Cadario & Chandon, 2018).

The appeal of this environmental approach to behavior change is that it might reach many people in a relatively low-cost manner. By simply rearranging products in a store or cafeteria, or by displaying some simple messages at the point of choice, dietary choices of (some) people may be influenced. Environmental interventions may work by decreasing exposure to high-calorie foods (e.g., by decreasing salience of such products in a store), such that learned stimulus response associations are less likely to guide behavior. Furthermore, informational messages at the point of choice may break more or less automatic psychological reactions to food (e.g., by inhibiting the hedonic goal of eating enjoyment) by activating a competing health goal (Papies & Hamstra, 2010). In this way these environmental nudges reduce the expression of the strongly learned unhealthy stimulus–response associations that make it hard for people to change their behavior.

However, there are also a number of interrelated problems with this behavior change approach from the perspective of consumers who would like to change their food consumption. First, for an individual consumer it is often not possible to change the food environment, except for example at home, or at the office. Because choices for food often occur in environments that are not under the control of a consumer (e.g., in the grocery store, in restaurants), the potential effect of changing the home or office environment alone (e.g., move high-calorie temptations out of sight) seems very limited. In addition, even when consumers could have more influence on the food environment, for instance, via policy regulations they can vote for, modifying the current food environment is not straightforward. For instance, policy makers have been criticized for being naïve by proposing environmental interventions to reduce consumption of high-energy foods, without considering how to still make a profit (e.g., advocating small portions whereas larger portions are more profitable; Wilson & Stolarz-Fantino, 2018). The economic goals of food producers and sellers (to maximize sales and profit) are often in conflict with the effects of environmental strategies of this type that reduce consumption. Thus, at this point in time it does not seem very realistic that sufficient changes in the food choice context will be implemented to support consumers who aim to reduce consumption of (high-calorie) foods.

Second, even when some parties would be willing to change the food environment, it seems unlikely that this environmental change is implemented across all food choice contexts people encounter (e.g., restaurants, grocery shops, refrigerator at home, cafeteria at work). This is problematic from a behavior change perspective, as effects of environmental interventions to change people's behavior tend to be constrained to the specific situation that is changed, and effects do not necessarily spill over to other contexts (Hertwig & Grüne-Yanoff, 2017). In other words, when we think about reducing choices for advertised HFSS products, and about reducing the quantity of consumption of such foods via environmental interventions, we need environmental changes across many situations and to make sure environments are not changed back. Finally, questions can be raised about the ethical aspects of environmental interventions to change people's behavior. The most effective environmental interventions are likely those in which certain options are forbidden, or hard to obtain, reducing people's freedom of choice.

Boosting behavior change

To address the problems raised above, recently a *boosting* approach to behavior change has been proposed (for elaborate conceptualizations, see Grüne-Yanoff & Hertwig, 2016; Hertwig & Grüne-Yanoff, 2017). The boosting approach focuses on providing people with competences that enable them to make decisions in line with their goals. The boosting approach addresses the problems discussed above in multiple ways. First, by focusing on people's competences rather than the environment as the target of intervention, this approach is suitable when implementing environmental changes is not straightforward, such as in the case of changing the food environment. Second, the advantage of focusing on competences is that, once a competence has been acquired, the competence can be helpful to change behavior across different relevant contexts. That is, once people learn to routinely select low- over high-calorie foods they can implement this skill whenever they are faced with such a choice. Third, the boosting approach emphasizes transparency and autonomy by teaching people competences that they can then use to change their own behavior in any way they like.

What would a boosting intervention to reduce intake of high-calorie foods look like? As explained earlier, one difficulty with inhibiting behavior toward advertised HFSS food is that this behavior is strongly guided by learned responses, which may lead to unintentional consumption of these foods. Therefore, recently researchers have started to develop cognitive training procedures to modify learned associations with food items (for a review, see Stice, Lawrence, Kemps, & Veling, 2016). The idea behind this approach is to couple the visual presentation of food items consistently with "moving away" avoidance reactions (e.g., Becker, Jostmann, Wiers, & Holland, 2015), or the inhibition of a motor response (called a "no-go" response; e.g., Veling et al., 2017), in order to break the strongly reinforced food-go responses. This in turn may change people's behavior toward the food items.

In the remaining part of this chapter we will discuss one specific cognitive training intervention, GNG training, which appears an effective means that people may use to reduce their consumption of high-calorie foods (for meta-analyses, see Allom, Mullan, & Hagger, 2015; Jones et al., 2016; Turton, Bruidegom, Cardi, Hirsch, & Treasure, 2016), and perhaps also to increase consumption of foods considered healthy. Although this training was originally not developed as a boosting intervention, it is interesting to view the training from this perspective. Specifically, as explained in more detail below, the training effectively reduces people's learned go responses to HFSS foods in general, and could be adapted to change responses to specific (favorite) brand products in particular, and may hence ultimately be offered to consumers as a tool they can use to change their behavior in the current food environment in any direction they wish. We will first explain the training procedure, and the main findings to date. Next, we present a first impression of an effort to turn this training procedure into a large-scale boosting intervention.

Modifying responses to food with GNG

GNG is a simple computerized training procedure in which images of food items, and sometimes images of non-food items, are presented one by one on a computer screen for around 1 second. Each item is consistently paired with either a cue to press a button (the go cue), or with a cue to withhold behavior (the no-go cue). The GNG cues can be auditory tones (e.g., high and low tones) or visual cues (e.g., thin or thick borders around the images). During GNG the amount of go (and no-go) trials is usually 50%, and the task is easy to perform because the cue is presented at the beginning of a trial and there is sufficient time to respond (often 1000 or 1500 ms; for a review, see Veling et al., 2017). People do not make many errors in this task. Some food items are consistently associated with no-go cues, and other food items, or non-food items, with go cues. So basically, people withhold their responses to some (unhealthy) food items (no-go food items), and they respond to other non-food items (go items), or other (healthy) foods (go-food items).

Research employing GNG has examined the effects of this training procedure on a number of measures. The most researched areas are effects of GNG on explicit food evaluation, food intake, food selection, and body weight. First, several experiments have shown that repeatedly not responding to food items decreases the evaluation of how attractive or liked these food items are as measured on explicit rating scales compared to both go-food items and food items not presented during GNG (untrained items; e.g., Chen, Veling, Dijksterhuis, & Holland, 2016; Chen, Veling, Dijksterhuis, & Holland, 2018; Lawrence, O'Sullivan, et al., 2015; Serfas, Florack, Büttner, & Voegeding, 2017).

Interestingly, evaluations of go-food items are sometimes, but not always, higher than untrained items (Chen et al., 2016). Thus, the task seems primarily effective in reducing evaluations of no-go items, which is called the no-go devaluation effect. To date, it is not entirely clear how no-go items are devalued, but it seems that this is not due to application of some sort of explicit rule that no-go items are bad. Instead, it seems more likely that not responding to food items during GNG may be accompanied by negative affect, perhaps due to an intrinsic association between response inhibition and negative affect, which becomes attached to the no-go food items (for more elaborate discussions, see Chen et al., 2016; Chen, Veling, Dijksterhuis, et al., 2018). In any case, an interesting feature of GNG is that it can make attractive food items less appealing.

Second, several studies have examined effects of GNG on food intake (Folkvord, Veling, & Hoeken, 2016; Houben & Jansen, 2011; Lawrence, Verbruggen, Morrison, Adams, & Chambers, 2015; Oomen, Grol, Spronk, Booth, & Fox, 2018; for a review, see Adams, Lawrence, Verbruggen, & Chambers, 2017). The first published study on food GNG training examined effects on chocolate intake (Houben & Jansen, 2011). Participants received a GNG task in which images of chocolate were consistently associated with no-go cues (chocolate no-go condition), or with go cues (chocolate go condition), or with both go and no-go cues (control condition). These different tasks were given to three different participant groups. Next, quantity of consumption was measured during a taste test. Results showed participants consumed less chocolate in the chocolate no-go condition compared to the control condition, while the go condition did not differ from both these conditions. Furthermore, the difference between the no-go chocolate condition and the other conditions was significantly stronger for participants who indicated that they are frequently dieting to lose weight. Other studies also suggest effects of GNG on intake might be stronger for people who score relatively high on dietary restraint (Lawrence, Verbruggen, et al., 2015; Veling, Aarts, & Papies, 2011).

One more recent study (Folkvord et al., 2016) examined whether GNG can be effective at reducing intake of advertised candy from a highly popular brand among children (age 7–10). In this study the children were first exposed to advertisements of a candy brand or a control advertisement. Next, one group of children received a GNG where the advertised products were presented with no-go cues and control objects (cute animals) with go cues. Another group received a control GNG where colored circles instead of the advertised products were presented on no-go trials. Subsequently, the children were asked to wait for a moment, and while they were waiting they had the opportunity to eat as much or as little candy as they liked. Two bowls were offered containing the advertised candy and another attractive brand of candy. Results showed that candy intake of both brands was substantially lower (more than 30%) among children who performed the GNG with the advertised products compared to the control group. Unlike some previous work, exposure to the candy advertisement did not increase candy intake compared to exposure to the control advertisement (Folkvord, Anschütz, Buijzen, & Valkenburg, 2013), perhaps because the advertisement was presented before the GNG, and immediate effects of advertisements on actual intake may wear off quickly.

In the research on food intake participants are generally presented with food to eat, and they do not choose the absolute portion or type of food themselves. Other research suggests that GNG can also influence the initial selection of food. First, research has shown that, when candies are repeatedly associated with no-go cues during GNG, participants select fewer of these candies to take home with them compared to when they performed a control task where they responded to these items, even when the GNG was performed 1 day before the food selection took place (Van Koningsbruggen, Veling, Stroebe, & Aarts, 2014, experiment 1). In another experiment the amount of candy participants received was contingent on how long they pressed a button, and participants pressed for a shorter time when candies had been presented with no-go cues (Van Koningsbruggen et al., 2014, experiment 2). Other research also suggests GNG decreases effort (i.e., amount of key presses) participants exert to obtain no-go food items (Houben & Giesen, 2018).

There is also work that examined effects of GNG on food choice. First, it has been shown that repeatedly not responding to some snack items decreases choices for these snack items compared to when participants responded to these snack items (Chen, Holland, Quandt, Dijksterhuis & Veling, 2019). This basic effect was replicated across multiple experiments, and this study also showed that a (weak) effect of the training on food choice was still visible 1 week after performing the training. Moreover, one experiment from this study showed GNG increased the probability of choosing a relatively nutritious food (vegetable or fruit) over HFSS food. Another study showed that 4–11-year-old children who were trained to consistently inhibit responding to energy-dense snack foods (and to respond to healthy foods) subsequently chose fewer energy-dense snacks, and more healthy snacks. This effect of training on healthier food choices was seen both relative to the children's choices before training (measured 5–10 days earlier) and relative to the choices of other children who were trained to either GNG to non-food items, or who were trained to inhibit responding to energy-dense snacks only half of the time (Porter et al., 2018).

Finally, work has examined whether GNG can be employed to facilitate weight loss attempts. In one of these experiments participants (mostly university students) were asked to perform a GNG online for 4 consecutive weeks (Veling, Koningsbruggen, Aarts, & Stroebe, 2014). One group received a GNG consisting of 100 food items that were all presented on no-go trials and 100 non-food control objects (all go). Another group received a GNG with non-foods presented on both go and no-go trials. Before and after the intervention participants' body weight was measured. Results showed that participants lost more weight when they received the GNG containing food images compared to the GNG containing non-food images only. This effect was stronger among participants with a relatively high body mass index.

Another study also compared the effects of online food with non-food GNG training on weight loss but this time in a sample of mostly overweight or obese middle-aged adults recruited from the community (Lawrence, O'Sullivan, et al., 2015). Participants had to complete four online GNG tasks in 1 week, with active participants being trained to no-go to nine energy-dense snack foods and to go to nine healthy foods, and control participants being trained to go and no-go to non-food items. Active, but not control, participants showed significant weight loss at 2-week and 6-month follow-up, reduced daily energy intake (calculated from food diaries), and reduced liking of the trained no-go foods.

In sum, GNG has been shown to reduce evaluations of no-go food items, and reduce intake of no-go foods, compared to conditions where this food was not presented during the training. Furthermore, GNG has been shown to influence the selection of food, and choices for food, such that people tend to select foods associated with go responses over foods associated with no-go responses. Finally, GNG has been shown to facilitate weight loss attempts among students and a community sample.

The mechanisms by which GNG changes people's responses to food are still under debate (e.g., Veling et al., 2017). One candidate mechanism is that GNG reduces the reward value of no-go food items, and thereby also more overt behaviors such as intake or choice. Another explanation is that GNG creates stimulus-go and stimulus-stop reactions which may respectively steer behavior toward or away from food. In any case, it seems plausible to assume that GNG changes people's learned affective and/or motor responses toward food, which may then subsequently facilitate behavior change. In the following section we will discuss to what degree the GNG might indeed be a helpful tool for consumers to change their responses to food in order to facilitate any behavior change they wish and overcome the negative effects of food marketing for unhealthy foods.

Turning GNG into a boost

To date, most work on effects of GNG has been examined in controlled environments such as the psychology laboratory. As a result, participants are not always informed about the possible effects of GNG on their behavior. In order to qualify as a boost, however, people should be informed about the possible effects of GNG on their behavior, so that they can decide whether or not to use this tool to modify their responses to food in a direction they wish (Hertwig & Grüne-Yanoff, 2017). Moreover, GNG has been mostly employed among university students who do not necessarily have the goal to change their responses to food (Stice et al., 2016). Hence, from a boosting perspective it is important to know whether GNG will still work when people intentionally use it as a tool to change their behavior.

Nonetheless, there are some indications in the literature reviewed above that GNG might have the potential to be turned into a boosting intervention. First, the GNG has been shown to facilitate weight loss attempts in two samples. In these studies, participants were informed that the GNG (in both the active and control conditions) might be helpful in facilitating weight loss. So, at least when it comes to these two weight loss studies, it seems that knowledge of the potential benefit of GNG does not fully negate any effects of this training. Of course it is still unclear whether this task still works when people are fully informed about what the task does and how it works (see also Lee, Dingle, Griffiths, & Lawrence, 2016).

Second, although GNG has mostly been studied with undergraduate students, GNG has also been shown to influence responses to food among children (Folkvord et al., 2016; Porter et al., 2018), a community sample (Lawrence, O'Sullivan, et al., 2015), and participants who are morbidly obese (Chen, Veling, De Vries, et al., 2018). These findings suggest that GNG may be useful to at least consider as the basis for a boosting intervention, as the task may be effective at changing responses to food among a wide variety of people.

In light of these considerations, recently a computer application has been developed that allows a wide dissemination of GNG to consumers. The training has recently been offered to the general public in a pragmatic open trial (Lawrence, Van Beurden, Javaid, & Mostazir, 2018). Both a web-delivered version of the training that works on desk-top computers (http://foodtraining. exeter.ac.uk/; used in the weight loss study by Lawrence, O'Sullivan et al., 2015) and a smartphone application (Food Trainer; available in the Apple and Android Play Store) have been used by over 100,000 people (the smartphone application alone has over 83,000 downloads). Preliminary analyses of data from more than 2000 users who provided complete data (pre-, training and post-training measures) suggest reductions in self-reported weight and frequency of intake of energy-dense snacks from before training to 4–6 weeks post-training. These reductions were larger for the web-delivered than the smartphone-delivered training, but unfortunately there is no control group to compare these reductions with. Several factors were associated with larger reductions in weight or snacking, including higher baseline body mass index and disinhibited (poorly controlled) eating scores, and completing a greater amount of training. Most participants reported that the training did or may have helped them to reduce their food intake and that they would or might recommend the intervention to a friend. These promising preliminary findings await validation in a large-scale randomized controlled trial with objective measures.

Nonetheless, some conclusions can already be drawn. First, at least tens of thousands of consumers seem interested in a smartphone application that modifies responses to food. This number may even increase when the smartphone app is advertised widely. Second, whilst a large number of people tried the training program, only a small proportion of them completed all of the pre- and post-training measures as part of the study. These measures were optional, but their relatively low completion, combined with the lack of a control group, means it is hard to get an accurate idea of the application's effects in the wider population.

Future directions

One important reason for engaging the public in this research on the online training app at an early stage has been to gather feedback about how the GNG training could be improved. Users have emphasized the need to personalize the training so that images of both go and no-go foods are tailored to their preferences and goals for dietary change (e.g., being trained to go to healthy foods that the user likes and can easily buy; and to no-go to items that represent strong temptations). The smartphone-application GNG training already includes some personalization, with users able to select no-go images from 15 categories of tempting energy-dense foods and drinks, and to select from five categories of healthy go foods. However, the personalization could be extended to allow users to incorporate their own photographs of foods and associated cues (e.g., foods in their branded packaging) into the training. Research is needed on whether such personalization will lead to stronger training effects.

Other research questions also remain to be addressed. First, it is unclear what the optimum number of foods is that individuals should train themselves to in order to maximize real-world changes in eating behavior. For instance, does the training work best when it is focused on particular kinds of foods such as sweet or savory snacks (e.g., Lawrence, O'Sullivan, et al., 2015), or is the training more effective when applied to a wider range of foods, including meals (e.g., Veling et al., 2014)?

Another key issue is the optimum frequency, timing, and duration of training. Users have found daily smartphone notifications useful to remind themselves to complete the training, but often report that effects dissipate when they stop doing the training regularly (Lawrence et al., 2018). It may take time for deeply engrained go responses to foods to be replaced by competing no-go ones in a sustained manner. Frequent repetition and practice of response inhibition to foods, in a wide range of contexts and at various times of day, may be required. Therefore, studies that manipulate the amount of training, how long it is continued for, and when it is done (at limited times of day and in specific places or across a broad range) would be helpful. Future studies should also take measures for a longer period of time to see how sustained the effects are (e.g., Chen et al., 2019).

Another important topic for future research is how best to measure training effects in large-scale trials. As indicated above, many people are unwilling to complete questionnaire measures and these are prone to bias (Schoeller et al., 2013). If we could capture changes in people's eating or food-purchasing behavior more "passively" (e.g., by accessing bank or store card statements) we might be able to measure effects of GNG training more objectively, accurately, and on a larger scale. Finally, some users report finding the training boring so research will need to determine whether gamifying the training by adding a more complex points system or speeding it up to make it more challenging will increase user engagement and enjoyment (Lumsden, Edwards, Lawrence, Coyle, & Munafò, 2016).

Conclusion

Many people are exposed to HFSS and meat products that are intensively promoted and advertised by large multinational companies. This makes sense from a commercial perspective, but this exposure can cause severe difficulties with (1) adhering to a healthy diet, and (2) intentionally changing daily dietary choices in a desired direction. In order to facilitate behavior change from HFSS and meat products toward lower-calorie nutritious plant-based foods that are not so heavily advertised (e.g., vegetables), the environment may be targeted such that it facilitates choices for these lower-calorie nutritious foods. Another approach would be to develop technological tools, such as smartphone apps, that enable consumers to change their learned associations with food in order to change their dietary choices in any direction they desire within the current food environment, for instance, away from heavily advertised HFSS and meat products. Which kind of approach will work best from a theoretical, applied, and pragmatic perspective remains to be seen in the coming years.

References

Adams, R. C., Lawrence, N. S., Verbruggen, F., & Chambers, C. D. (2017). Training response inhibition to reduce food consumption: Mechanisms, stimulus specificity and appropriate training protocols. *Appetite, 109*, 11–23.

Allom, V., Mullan, B., & Hagger, M. (2015). Does inhibitory control training improve health behaviour? A meta-analysis. *Health Psychology Review, 10*(2), 168–186.

Andreyeva, T., Kelly, I. R., & Harris, J. L. (2011). Exposure to food advertising on television: Associations with children's fast food and soft drink consumption and obesity. *Economics & Human Biology, 9*(3), 221–233.

Becker, D., Jostmann, N. B., Wiers, R. W., & Holland, R. W. (2015). Approach avoidance training in the eating domain: Testing the effectiveness across three single session studies. *Appetite, 85*, 58–65.

Berridge, K. C. (2009). 'Liking' and 'wanting' food rewards: Brain substrates and roles in eating disorders. *Physiology & Behavior, 97*, 537–550.

Berridge, K. C., & Robinson, T. E. (2003). Parsing reward. *Trends in Neuroscience, 26*, 507–513.

Boswell, R. G., & Kober, H. (2016). Food cue reactivity and craving predict eating and weight gain: A meta-analytic review. *Obesity Reviews, 17*, 159–177.

Brester, G. W., & Schroeder, T. C. (1995). The impacts of brand and generic advertising on meat demand. *American Journal of Agricultural Economics, 77*(4), 969–979.

Brownell, K. D., Farley, T., Willett, W. C., Popkin, B. M., Chaloupka, F. J., Thompson, J. W., & Ludwig, D. S. (2009). The public health and economic benefits of taxing sugar-sweetened beverages. *The New England Journal of Medicine, 15*, 1599–1605.

Cadario, R., & Chandon, P. (2018). Which healthy eating nudges work best? A meta-analysis of field experiments. *Marketing Science* (forthcoming). Retrieved from: http://dx.doi.org/10.2139/ssrn.3090829

Carter, P., Bignardi, G., Hollands, G. J., & Marteau, T. (2018). BMC Public Health: Information-based cues at point of choice to change selection and consumption of food, alcohol and tobacco products: A systematic review. *BMC Public Health, 18*(1), 418. Retrieved from: https://doi.org/10.17863/CAM.22472

Chen, Z., Holland, R. W., Quandt, J., Dijksterhuis, A., & Veling, H. (2019). When mere action versus inaction leads to robust preference change. *Journal of Personality and Social Psychology* doi: 10.1037/pspa0000158.

Chen, Z., Veling, H., De Vries, S. P., Bijvank, B. O., Janssen, I. M. C., Dijksterhuis, A., & Holland, R. W. (2018). Go/no-go training changes food evaluation in both morbidly obese and normal-weight individuals. *Journal of Consulting and Clinical Psychology*, *86*(12), 980–990.

Chen, Z., Veling, H., Dijksterhuis, A., & Holland, R. W. (2016). How does not responding to appetitive stimuli cause devaluation: Evaluative conditioning or response inhibition? *Journal of Experimental Psychology: General*, *145*, 1687–1701. http://dx.doi.org/10.1037/xge0000236

Chen, Z., Veling, H., Dijksterhuis, A., & Holland, R. W. (2018). Do impulsive individuals benefit more from food go/no-go training? Testing the role of inhibition capacity in the no-go devaluation effect. *Appetite*, *124*, 99–110.

Dorresteijn, J. A., Van der Graaf, Y., Zheng, K., Spiering, W., & Visseren, F. L. (2013). The daily 10 kcal expenditure deficit: a before-and-after study on low-cost interventions in the work environment. *BMJ Open*, *3*(1), e002125.

Elfhag, K., & Rössner, S. (2005). Who succeeds in maintaining weight loss? A conceptual review of factors associated with weight loss maintenance and weight regain. *Obesity Reviews*, *6*(1), 67–85.

Epstein, L. H., Carr, K. A., Lin, H., & Fletcher, K. D (2011). Food reinforcement, energy intake, and macronutrient choice. *American Journal of Clinical Nutrition*, *94*, 12–18.

Folkvord, F., Anschütz, D. J., Buijzen, M., & Valkenburg, P. M. (2013). The effect of playing advergames that promote energy-dense snacks or fruit on actual food intake among children. *The American Journal of Clinical Nutrition*, *97*, 239–245.

Folkvord, F., Veling, H., & Hoeken, H. (2016). Targeting implicit approach reactions to snack food in children: Effects on snack intake. *Health Psychology*, *35*, 919–922.

Freeman, S. M., Razhas, I., & Aron, A. R. (2014). Top-down response suppression mitigates action tendencies triggered by a motivating stimulus. *Current Biology*, *24*(2), 212–216.

Friese, M., Wänke, M., & Plessner, H. (2006). Implicit consumer preferences and their influence on product choice. *Psychology & Marketing*, *23*(9), 727–740.

Grüne-Yanoff, T., & Hertwig, R. (2016). Nudge versus boost: How coherent are policy and theory? *Minds and Machines*, *26*(1–2), 149–183.

Hertwig, R., & Grüne-Yanoff, T. (2017). Nudging and boosting: Steering or empowering good decisions. *Perspectives on Psychological Science*, *12*, 973–986.

Holden, S. S., Zlatevska, N., & Dubelaar, C. (2016). Whether smaller plates reduce consumption depends on who's serving and who's looking: A meta-analysis. *Journal of the Association for Consumer Research*, *1*(1), 134–146.

Hollands, G. J., Bignardi, G., Johnston, M., Kelly, M. P., Ogilvie, D., Petticrew, M., . . . & Marteau, T. M. (2017). The TIPPME intervention typology for changing environments to change behaviour. *Nature Human Behaviour*, *1*(8), 0140.

Houben, K., & Giesen, J. C. (2018). Will work less for food: Go/no-go training decreases the reinforcing value of high-caloric food. *Appetite*, *130*, 79–83.

Houben, K., & Jansen, A. (2011). Training inhibitory control. A recipe for resisting sweet temptations. *Appetite*, *56*, 345–349.

Jones, A., Di Lemma, L., Robinson, E., Christiansen, P., Nolan, S., Tudur-Smith, C., & Field, M. (2016). Inhibitory control training for appetitive behaviour change: A meta-analytic investigation of mechanisms of action and moderators of effectiveness. *Appetite*, *97*, 16–28.

Lawrence, N. S., O'Sullivan, J., Parslow, D. M., Javaid, M., Adams, R. C., Chambers, C. D., Kos, K., Verbruggen, F. (2015). Training response inhibition to food is associated with weight loss and reduced calorie intake. *Appetite*, *95*, 17–28.

Lawrence, N. S., Van Beurden, S., Javaid, M., & Mostazir, M. M. (2018). Mass dissemination of web and smartphone-delivered food response inhibition training to reduce unhealthy snacking. *Appetite*, *130*, 309.

Lawrence, N. S., Verbruggen, F., Morrison, S., Adams, R. C., & Chambers, C. D. (2015). Stopping to food can reduce intake: Effects of stimulus-specificity and individual differences in dietary restraint. *Appetite*, *85*, 91–103.

Lee, R., Dingle, K., Griffiths, E., & Lawrence, N. (2016). Explicit and implicit training of food response inhibition is associated with food devaluation and weight loss. *Appetite*, *107*, 686.

Lumsden, J., Edwards, E. A., Lawrence, N. S., Coyle, D., & Munafò, M. R. (2016). Gamification of cognitive assessment and cognitive training: A systematic review of applications and efficacy. *JMIR Serious Games*, *4*(2).

Oomen, D., Grol, M., Spronk, D., Booth, C., & Fox, E. (2018). Beating uncontrolled eating: Training inhibitory control to reduce food intake and food cue sensitivity. *Appetite*, *131*, 73–83.

Papies, E. K., & Hamstra, P. (2010). Goal priming and eating behavior: Enhancing self-regulation by environmental cues. *Health Psychology*, *29*, 384–388.

Papies, E. K., & Veling, H. (2013). Healthy dining. Subtle diet reminders at the point of purchase increase low-calorie food choices among both chronic and current dieters. *Appetite*, *61*, 1–7.

Porter, L., Bailey-Jones, C., Priudokaite, G., Allen, S., Wood, K., Stiles, K., . . . Lawrence, N. S. (2018). From cookies to carrots; the effect of inhibitory control training on children's snack selections. *Appetite*, *124*, 111–123.

Rangel, A. (2013). Regulation of dietary choice by the decision-making circuitry. *Nature Neuroscience*, *16*(12), 1717–1724.

Robinson, T. N., Borzekowski, D. L., Matheson, D. M., & Kraemer, H. C. (2007). Effects of fast food branding on young children's taste preferences. *Archives of Pediatrics & Adolescent Medicine*, *161*, 792–797.

Rozin, P., Markwith, M., & Stoess, C. (1997). Moralization and becoming a vegetarian: The transformation of preferences into values and the recruitment of disgust. *Psychological Science*, *8*(2), 67–73.

Rozin, P., & Zellner, D. (1985). The role of pavlovian conditioning in the acquisition of food likes and dislikes. *Annals of the New York Academy of Sciences*, *443*(1), 189–202.

Santos, I., Sniehotta, F. F., Marques, M. M., Carraça, E. V., & Teixeira, P. J. (2017). Prevalence of personal weight control attempts in adults: A systematic review and meta-analysis. *Obesity Reviews*, *18*, 32–50.

Schoeller, D. A., Thomas, D., Archer, E., Heymsfield, S. B., Blair, S. N., Goran, M. I., . . . & Dhurandhar, N. V. (2013). Self-report-based estimates of energy intake offer an inadequate basis for scientific conclusions. *The American Journal of Clinical Nutrition*, *97*(6), 1413–1415.

Serfas, B. G., Florack, A., Büttner, O. B., & Voegeding, T. (2017). What does it take for sour grapes to remain sour? Persistent effects of behavioral inhibition in go/no-go tasks on the evaluation of appetitive stimuli. *Motivation Science*, *3*(1), 1.

Stice, E., Lawrence, N. S., Kemps, E., & Veling, H. (2016). Training motor responses to food: A novel treatment for obesity targeting implicit processes. *Clinical Psychology Review*, *49*, 16–27.

Story, M., & French, S. (2004). Food advertising and marketing directed at children and adolescents in the US. *International Journal of Behavioral Nutrition and Physical Activity*, *1*(1), 3.

Strack, F., & Deutsch, R. (2004). Reflective and impulsive determinants of social behavior. *Personality and Social Psychology Review*, *8*(3), 220–247.

Stroebe, W., Van Koningsbruggen, G. M., Papies, E. K., & Aarts, H. (2013). Why most dieters fail but some succeed: A goal conflict model of eating behavior. *Psychological Review*, *120*(1), 110–138.

Sullivan, N., Hutcherson, C., Harris, A., & Rangel, A. (2015). Dietary self-control is related to the speed with which attributes of healthfulness and tastiness are processed. *Psychological science*, *26*(2), 122–134.

Thaler, R., & Sunstein, C. R. (2008). *Nudge: Improving decisions about health, wealth and happiness*. New York, NY: Simon & Schuster.

Thorndike, A. N., Riis, J., Sonnenberg, L. M., & Levy, D. E. (2014). Traffic-light labels and choice architecture: Promoting healthy food choices. *American Journal of Preventive Medicine*, *46*, 143–149.

Turton, R., Bruidegom, K., Cardi, V., Hirsch, C. R., & Treasure, J. (2016). Novel methods to help develop healthier eating habits for eating and weight disorders: A systematic review and meta-analysis. *Neuroscience & Biobehavioral Reviews*, *61*, 132–155.

Van den Akker, K., Schyns, G., & Jansen, A. (2018). Learned overeating: Applying principles of pavlovian conditioning to explain and treat overeating. *Current Addiction Reports*, *5*, 223–231.

Van Gucht, D., Vansteenwegen, D., Van den Bergh, O., & Beckers, T. (2008). Conditioned craving cues elicit an automatic approach tendency. *Behaviour Research and Therapy*, *46*(10), 1160–1169.

Van Koningsbruggen, G. M., Veling, H., Stroebe, W., & Aarts, H. (2014). Comparing two psychological interventions in reducing impulsive processes of eating behaviour: Effects on self-selected portion size. *British Journal of Health Psychology*, *19*, 767–782.

Veling, H., Aarts, H., & Papies, E. K. (2011). Using stop signals to inhibit chronic dieters' responses toward palatable foods. *Behaviour Research & Therapy*, *49*, 771–780.

Veling, H., Koningsbruggen, G., Aarts, H., & Stroebe, W. (2014). Targeting impulsive processes of eating behavior via the internet. Effects on body weight. *Appetite*, *78*, 102–109.

Veling, H., Lawrence, N. S., Chen, Z., Van Koningsbruggen, G. M., & Holland, R. W. (2017). What is trained during food go/no-go training? A review focusing on mechanisms and a research agenda. *Current Addiction Reports*, *4*(1), 35–41.

Watson, P., Wiers, R. W., Hommel, B., & De Wit, S. (2014). Working for food you don't desire. Cues interfere with goal-directed food-seeking. *Appetite*, *79*, 139–148.

Watson, P., Wiers, R. W., Hommel, B., Gerdes, V. E., & de Wit, S. (2017). Stimulus control over action for food in obese versus healthy-weight individuals. *Frontiers in Psychology*, *8*, 580.

Wilfley, D. E., Hayes, J. F., Balantekin, K. N., Van Buren, D. J., & Epstein, L. H. (2018). Behavioral interventions for obesity in children and adults: Evidence base, novel approaches, and translation into practice. *American Psychologist*, *73*(8), 981.

Wilson, A. L., Buckley, E., Buckley, J. D., & Bogomolova, S. (2016). Nudging healthier food and beverage choices through salience and priming. Evidence from a systematic review. *Food Quality and Preference*, *51*, 47–64.

Wilson, B. M., & Stolarz-Fantino, S. (2018). Bundling the way to bankruptcy: Economic theory should inform the design of sugary-drink menus used in research. *Psychological Science*, *29*(8), 1376–1379.

7

THE PROMOTION OF HEALTHY FOODS

A review of the literature and theoretical framework

Dr. Frans Folkvord

Introduction

Current dietary intake of children and adolescents is poor and does not meet (inter) national nutritional standards (Karnik & Kanekar, 2012; Mackenbach et al., 2008; Willett et al., 2019). As a consequence of this unhealthy eating pattern, we are currently facing a global epidemic of childhood obesity and, in line with this trend, non-communicable diseases that are highly related to dietary intake and which are relatively easy to prevent. Considering that unhealthy eating patterns develop during childhood and continue into adolescence and adulthood, this trend is very likely to accelerate in decades to come (Lobstein et al., 2015).

The World Health Organization (WHO) has stated recently, and has in fact been reiterating continuously for decades, that prevention and treatment of childhood obesity are among the highest priorities (Lobstein et al., 2015; WHO, 2017). Together with an increasing number of researchers, health institutes, non-governmental organizations, parents, and primary and secondary school teachers and principals, the WHO argues that more needs to be done to improve dietary intake of young children. For example, celebrity chef Jamie Oliver, who has conducted multiple large intervention projects to improve dietary intake among children from different age groups across countries by actively promoting healthier foods, has found it to be extremely difficult to improve eating behaviors of children. This holds in particular for those living in low-socioeconomic-status geographical areas, and even applies in his native country, the United Kingdom. Here, Oliver is immensely popular and one would assume a certain impact would spill forth from his efforts. The health benefits related to the intake of healthy foods, such as fruit and vegetables, are very well known and studies by a great variety of international researchers have shown this extensively over many decades. Unfortunately, actual intake is still lacking with respect to international recommendations.

Obesogenic context

One important factor that explains the unhealthy eating patterns of people, and children in particular, is the context in which they live and consume their foods. The so-called "obesogenic" environment, defined as the accumulation of influences that the surrounding opportunities, or conditions of life, have on promoting obesity in individuals or populations (Lake & Townshend, 2006), promotes and stimulates the consumption of energy-dense foods over healthier foods, in contrast to the repeated recommendations of health practitioners (Pearce et al., 2009; Swinburn, Egger, & Raza, 1999).

Although not all factors influencing eating behavior are easy to modify, some, in fact, are. For example, environment and food-related experiences have consistently been shown to be central to the development of children's eating behavior (Birch, 1999). Central to understanding how parents, their environments, and wider structural contexts might affect and shape children's current and long-term eating behavior is gaining insight in how preferences, attitudes, and food choices are shaped through the promotion of foods in the near environment (DeCosta, Møller, Frøst, & Olsen, 2017), which I will discuss in the rest of this chapter.

A great number of studies have shown that the intake of fruits and vegetables among children lies decidedly below recommended guidelines (Spence, Campbell, Lioret, & McNaughton, 2018; Willett et al., 2019). Because dietary patterns of children and adolescents continue into adulthood, targeting children's fruit and vegetable intake improves healthy lifestyles across the life span and has a strong effect on non-communicable diseases and mental well-being (Kaikkonen et al.,; Lobstein et al., 2015; Swinburn et al., 1999). Therefore, motivating and inducing children to eat more fruit and vegetables will regain and maintain healthy weight statuses and also improve other health indicators (e.g., inflammation levels, blood lipids, blood pressure, insulin sensitivity, mental well-being: Lock, Pomerleau, Causer, Altmann, & McKee, 2005; Ness & Powles, 1997; Willett, 1994). In addition, the intake of fruit and vegetables is negatively related to overweight and obesity (Spear et al., 2007), psychological dysfunctioning (Rooney, McKinley, & Woodside, 2013), risk of cardiovascular disease (Bazzano et al., 2002), coronary heart disease and hypertension (Joshipura et al., 2001), and multiple forms of cancer (Aune et al., 2017). Considering that a large part of the world's population is inadequately nourished and many environmental systems and processes are pushed beyond safe boundaries by the current levels of food consumption, a global transformation of what people eat is urgently needed (Willett et al., 2019).

The current chapter describes recent findings regarding the effects of food promotion techniques of healthy foods among children and their effect on eating behavior, as well as integrating these empirical findings in a new theoretical framework that can be used for future research in this area.

Hedonic foods

In general, high-fat, sugar, and sodium foods such as pizzas, French fries, candy, and chocolate are experienced as intrinsically rewarding. As a result, such foods contain more intrinsic motivational capacities and incentive qualities than healthier foods such as fruit and vegetables, giving shape to unhealthy eating habits (Berridge & Kringelbach, 2015; Berridge & Robinson, 2003). This unhealthy dietary intake pattern is found in most Western countries, and increasingly in the rest of the world, thereby affecting both physical and mental health on a global level (Vandevijvere, Chow, Hall, Umali, & Swinburn, 2015). Worth mentioning in this context is that, over the past few decades, countries that are well known for having a more traditional cuisine, Italy and France serving as prime examples, have also been seen to shift towards the intake of more processed and energy-dense foods instead of the Mediterranean diet and *haute cuisine* that have been key elements of their respective cultures.

The motivation to consume energy-dense foods is however not only based on the intrinsic properties of food products. The reinforcing value and consumption of food are also stimulated by way of external cues, predominantly through a large variation of food promotion techniques (as we have seen in other chapters in this volume). Food companies create messages to prime children to focus on the hedonic aspects of food, in this way directing their attention more on the liking and wanting of specific food items and inducing unhealthy eating behavior (Boyland et al., 2016; Cairns, Angus, Hastings, & Caraher, 2013; Folkvord, Anschütz, Boyland, Kelly, & Buijzen, 2016; Folkvord, Anschütz, Buijzen, & Valkenburg, 2013; Folkvord, Anschütz, Nederkoorn, Westerik, & Buijzen, 2014; Folkvord, Anschütz, Wiers, & Buijzen, 2015). This mechanism improves the attitudes and perceptions of these (unhealthy) foods, increasing the probability that recipients of such messages are motivated to consume the advertised foods. Numerous behavioral models, such as dual-process models and cue reactivity theory, propose that eating behavior is only to a limited extent guided by a conscious, reflective, rule-based system, and more dominantly via a non-conscious, impulsive, associative system (Folkvord, Veling, & Hoeken, 2016; Hofmann, Rauch, & Gawronski, 2007; Papies, 2016; Sheeran, Gollwitzer, & Bargh, 2013).

Until now, studies examining food promotion activities have predominantly focused on the marketing of energy-dense foods (Boyland et al., 2016; Folkvord, Anschütz, et al., 2016). Many researchers and international experts have concluded that food promotion results in effective modification of attitudes, affections, intentions, and, ultimately, consumption behavior (Boswell & Kober, 2016; Boyland & Halford, 2013; Boyland et al., 2016; Folkvord, Anschütz, et al., 2016; Galbraith-Emami & Lobstein, 2013). Despite the introduction of government regulations and industry codes of practice for responsible food promotion, recent content analysis of food-related promotion on television shows that food marketing primarily directed at minors still predominantly promotes unhealthy food products (Harris, LoDolce, Dembek, & Schwartz, 2015; Norman et al., 2018).

Modifying external values

Currently, increasing attention is being paid to modifying children's eating behavior in a more desirable direction. From a political, societal, and public health perspective, this is undoubtedly due to the rise in childhood obesity rates and the concerns relating to the long-term health consequences that this rise may have. This rise in childhood obesity is worrying not only in connection with the increased risk of non-communicable diseases with which these children are faced at an early age, but also, and even more importantly, because dietary intake during childhood continues into adolescence and adulthood.

Given the effectiveness and success of food promotion of unhealthy foods, it might be a highly promising avenue to investigate *whether, how, when*, and *for whom* food promotion techniques of healthy foods increase the reinforcing value of foods such as fruit and vegetables. As a consequence of increased reinforcing value, such exposure might subsequently also increase the intake of these foods among children (De Droog, Buijzen & Valkenburg, 2014; Folkvord, Anasatasiadou, & Anschütz, 2017; Folkvord, Veling, et al., 2016; Hanks, Just, & Brumberg, 2016; Rangel, 2013). To arrive at an overarching theoretical model that explains and predicts how food promotion of healthier foods might be effective, an extensive synthesis of existing theoretical models from different disciplines and a review of recent empirical evidence were conducted.

The Promotion of Healthy Food Model

The proposed theoretical model contains an eclectic combination of theories from research fields that have studied eating behavior from different angles for decades (i.e., consumer psychology, developmental psychology, biology, neuroscience, sociology, nutritional science, behavioral economics, and communication science). Integrating findings from such differing research fields leads to important insights on how to stimulate, for example, children's fruit and vegetable intake, which can be used for research and practice in a variety of disciplines.

The five foundational assumptions of the *Promotion of Healthy Food Model* (Figure 7.1) are that: (1) by increasing attention toward, and the reinforcing value (e.g., liking and wanting) of fruit and vegetables through food promotion, (2) a reciprocal relation with eating behavior occurs, which in time (3) leads to a normalization of intake of fruit and vegetables (habit formation) and, ultimately, (4) to improved health states as indicated by physiological (e.g., inflammation levels, blood lipids, blood pressure, insulin sensitivity, neurological activity, weight) and psychological (e.g., craving, hunger, general well-being) improvements. Furthermore, (5) individual and societal factors (e.g., impulsivity, body mass index, gender, socioeconomic status, food fussiness, parental feeding style) determine susceptibility to food promotion. In the next section, we will explain the Promotion of Healthy Food Model in more detail.

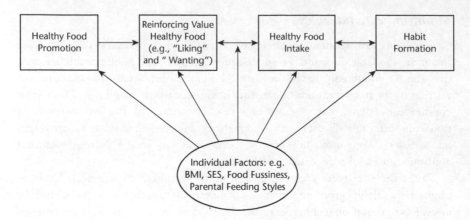

FIGURE 7.1 The Promotion of Healthy Foods Model. BMI, body mass intake; SES, socioeconomic status.

The effect of food promotion on reinforcing value and intake

In addition to homeostatic signals or habits, eating behavior is stimulated through hedonic influences and by the reinforcing value of foods (e.g., liking and wanting; Berridge & Kringelbach, 2015; Berridge & Robinson, 2003). For example, the cue reactivity theory (Carter & Tiffany, 1999) and Reactivity to Embedded Food Cues in Advertising Model (REFCAM; Folkvord, Anschütz, et al., 2016) propose that food cues in promotional activities trigger a number of physiological responses, such as increased heart rate, gastric activity, and salivation (Nederkoorn, Smulders, & Jansen, 2000), and heightened activation of the dopaminergic reward system (Nijs, Franken, & Muris, 2010; Volkow, Wang, Fowler, & Telang, 2008). In addition, several psychological responses such as increased attention for food-related cues (Folkvord, Anschütz, et al. 2016; Nijs et al., 2010; Nijs, Muris, Euser, & Franken, 2010) and cravings and thoughts about food intake (Berridge & Robinson, 2003; Boon, Stroebe, Schut, & Jansen, 1998; Carter & Tiffany, 1999; Kakoschke, Kemps, & Tiggemann, 2014; Provencher, Polivy, & Herman, 2009) are triggered.

With frequency and duration of exposure, internal and external stimuli (the conditioned stimulus) become associated with the rewarding foods (unconditioned stimulus) through pavlovian conditioning (Berridge & Robinson, 2003; Carter & Tiffany, 1999). For example, several functional neuroimaging studies have shown that the nucleus accumbens, part of the dopaminergic reward pathway of the brain and considered as the functional interface between motivational food cues and consumption behaviors (Zahm, 2000), is activated in response to food advertisements (Rapuano et al., 2017; Rapuano, Huckins, Sargent, Heatherton, & Kelley, 2015).

As a consequence of the created associations between external cues and food intake, conditioned stimuli come to elicit activation of a central appetitive state, resulting in eating behavior responses (Berridge & Robinson, 2003; Carter & Tiffany, 1999; Volkow et al., 2008). Presenting and priming children more often with cues of fruit and vegetables by increasing their availability and presence, for example, could affect children into consuming more healthier foods in a more automatic way – importantly, bypassing deliberate choice-making processes (Berridge & Kringelbach, 2015; Fisher, Nicholas, & Marshall, 2011; Forwood, Ahern, Hollands, Ng, & Marteau, 2015; Kakoschke et al., 2014; Shepherd et al., 2006; Stevenson, Doherty, Barnett, Muldoon, & Trew, 2007). When, via food promotion techniques, healthier foods in this way attain an increased rewarding effect on a psychological and physiological level, this could strengthen the connection between exposure to, and subsequent intake of, fruit and vegetables (Chandon & Wansink, 2012; Cooke et al., 2011).

If promotional techniques manage to address young people's emotional and cognitive needs for identity and belonging, they can increase the rewarding attributes of fruit and vegetables (Bruce et al., 2013; De Cock, Van Lippevelde, Goossen et al., 2016; Folkvord, Anschütz, et al., 2016; Pempek & Calvert, 2009). For example, studies have repeatedly shown (Baldassarre & Campo, 2015; De Droog, Valkenburg, & Buijzen, 2010; De Droog et al., 2014) that using brand characters to promote fruit increases intake among children. Furthermore, a recent study has found that branded media dramatically increased children's vegetable selection (Hanks et al., 2016).

Other studies have found that stimulating fruit intake among children via advergames (Pempek & Calvert, 2009) or memory games (Folkvord et al., 2017) increases fruit intake, but a similar effect was not found for vegetables (Folkvord & Laguna-Camacho, 2019). Due to the intake and rewarding experience, reactivity to food-related cues becomes a stronger predictor of subsequent food intake (Rangel, 2013), and an increased food intake in turn reinforces the reactivity to food cues, resulting in the stimulation of a reciprocal relation between cued reactivity and food intake. This mechanism has previously been identified as the incentive–sensitization process (Berridge & Kringelbach, 2015; Berridge & Robinson, 2003; Boyland et al., 2016; Folkvord, Anschütz, et al., 2016) and could also be applicable to fruit and vegetables.

The current theoretical model shows that it is important to motivate children to want the foods (e.g., positive attitude, intention to buy and consume, preference over other foods, hedonic response (liking), willingness to taste), because food types that have high energy content but low nutritional value (e.g., energy-dense snacks) are more often considered, both physiologically and psychologically, as rewarding than food types that have low energy content but high nutritional value (e.g., fruit and vegetables). Currently, the first are consumed excessively while the latter are consumed insufficiently, resulting in a poor diet quality (Karnik & Kanekar, 2012; WHO, 2017) and subsequent poor health, both physiological and psychological.

Improving long-term health by habit formation

Repeated consumption of fruit and vegetables is essential in the creation of new habits. First, numerous studies have shown that repeatedly exposing and tasting fruit and vegetables increases their liking, thereby increasing the likelihood that they will be consumed in the future (Anzman-Frasca, Savage, Marini, Fisher, & Birch, 2012; Caton et al., 2014). Second, if exposure and tasting of fruit and vegetables increase, the behavior and taste become internalized in children (Papies, 2016; van't Riet, Sijtsema, Dagevos, & de Bruijn, 2011). Consequently, children will more likely integrate fruit and vegetables into their daily eating behavior, habitualizing the consumption of fruit and vegetables and thereby possibly substituting the unhealthy snacks with healthier snacks (Alissa & Ferns, 2017; Papies, 2016; van't Riet et al., 2011).

The great importance of studying long-term effects is that they are necessary for establishing vital health improvements, in particular among children (Alissa & Ferns, 2017; Karnik & Kanekar, 2012; Papies, 2016; van't Riet et al., 2011; WHO, 2017). For example, some studies have shown that healthier diets are associated with favorable changes in a range of cardiovascular disease risk markers, including continuous decreases in blood lipids and blood pressure, body weight and fat mass, and favorable changes in the homeostatic system (Sandström, Marckmann, & Bindslev, 1992; Szymlek-Gay, Ferguson, Heath, Gray, & Gibson, 2009). Short-term focused manipulations are of high value in order to reveal whether these manipulations are effective in inducing healthy foods, but healthy eating habits in children can only be formed when they are repeatedly and intensively exposed to the promotion of healthy foods.

For now, it remains unclear whether the promotion of healthier foods will also result in sustainable healthy eating habits. That is, most studies have only examined immediate or short-term effects of healthy food promotion techniques (Baldassarre & Campo, 2015, De Droog et al., 2010, 2014; Dovey, Taylor, Stow, Boyland, & Halford, 2011; Folkvord et al., 2017). Therefore, longitudinal studies are needed that go beyond these temporary effects and examine the effects of prolonged food promotion that can foster habitual behavior concerning fruit and vegetable intake.

Individual and contextual susceptibility

Multiple individual and contextual factors have been identified that can explain susceptibility to food promotion of unhealthy foods (Folkvord, Anschütz, et al., 2016; Valkenburg and Peter, 2013). For example, gender (Anschutz, Engels, & van Strien, 2009, 2010), impulsivity (Folkvord et al., 2014), weight status (Halford et al., 2008), and attentional bias (Folkvord et al., 2015) have all been found to moderate the effect of unhealthy food promotion on children's intake (Folkvord et al., 2016). But whether these concepts moderate the effect of promotion of fruit and vegetables has not been examined. Children who were found to be more impulsive (Folkvord et al., 2014) or had an attentional bias for foods (Folkvord et al., 2015) were more strongly influenced by food advertising of unhealthy foods than children who were less impulsive or did not have an attentional bias relating to foods. If food promotion techniques for fruit and vegetables can attract the attention of children, it might be the case that these latter groups of children are more susceptible to such effects as well.

Other individual factors that are recognized as possibly moderating are food neophobia (Dovey et al., 2011), food fussiness (Fildes, van Jaarsveld, Cooke, Wardle, & Llewellyn, 2016), and food knowledge (Boyland, Kavanagh-Safran, & Halford, 2015). Additionally, contextual factors such as where the food promotional techniques are shown (e.g., in school: Langford et al., 2017), parental feeding techniques (Carnell, Benson, Driggin, & Kolbe, 2014), or socioeconomic status (Shrewsbury & Wardle, 2008) are strongly related to the intake of fruit and vegetables. Establishing these, and other, individual and contextual dispositional factors is vital for two reasons: (1) for a new theoretical model that may explain future findings, and (2) in understanding the variability in the processing of the promotion of fruit and vegetables, the attention for, and reinforcing value of, these foods, as well as subsequent intake.

Guidelines for future research

The Promotion of Healthy Food Model explains recent empirical findings and aims to stimulate new scientific research in order to improve dietary intake among children.

First, the exact mechanisms underlying the effects of fruit and vegetable food promotion on actual intake have not been addressed adequately up until recently, and need further examination. One important line of inquiry could, for example, examine whether the promotion of fruit and vegetables influences actual craving, by studying physiological and psychological responses that prepare children for future intake, such as increased saliva or food intake-related hormones (e.g., insulin, ghrelin), or instead affects thoughts and motivations about the intake of food when children are exposed to these promotional techniques (Folkvord, Anschütz, et al., 2016).

Ferriday and Brunstrom (2011) have shown that adults with obesity show increased salivary responses and craving after exposure to unhealthy food cues compared to adults with normal weight, but this effect has not been studied extensively for healthier types of food. Others have shown that people with the fat mass and obesity-associated gene had greater caloric consumption after food advertisement exposure than people without this genotype (Gilbert-Diamond, Li, Adachi-Mejia, McClure, & Sargent, 2014). In addition, it would be interesting to examine if brain areas relating to the reward system are activated when children are exposed to the promotion of fruit and vegetables (Bruce et al., 2013; Gearhardt, Yokum, Stice, Harris, & Brownell, 2014; Volkow, Wang, & Baler, 2011), and if this consequently increases the actual intake of these foods because of the intensified rewarding value. Previous studies have found an effect of the promotion of healthy foods on intake among children (Baldassarre & Campo, 2015, De Droog et al., 2010, 2014;

Dovey et al., 2011; Folkvord et al., 2017; Just & Price, 2013), and several studies have found a neurological effect of food advertising for unhealthy foods in children (Bruce et al., 2013; Gearhardt et al., 2014; Zahm, 2000), but this has not yet been tested for promotion techniques for healthy foods. For example, Gearhardt et al. (2014) have shown that adolescents exhibited greater activation in regions implicated in reward areas during exposure to unhealthy food promotions, but this effect has not yet been tested using healthy food promotions and could be very informative in this line of research.

Second, future research should examine whether and how the accumulation of food promotion techniques for healthy foods influences the classical and operant conditioning of food cues and subsequent intake of healthier foods among children. The proposed theoretical model considers the effects of food promotion techniques on food intake (via cue reactivity) as a process of classical and operant conditioning, but it is as yet unclear what the long-term effects of food promotion techniques of healthy food are and whether they lead to improved health indicators. Whereas most of the studies reported above focused on fruit and vegetable intake, the model can also be applied for other foods that are considered to be healthy (water, legumes, nuts, and whole grains, to name but a few).

Third, although multiple individual (e.g., body mass index, impulsivity, attentional bias, neophobia, food fussiness) and contextual factors (e.g., socioeconomic status, parental feeding techniques) have been investigated that affect the influence of food promotion of unhealthy foods on eating behavior (Folkvord, Anschütz, et al., 2016), it remains unclear if these factors moderate the effect of promotion of healthy foods. Establishing these, and other, individual and contextual dispositional factors is vital for two reasons: (1) for a new theoretical model that may explain future findings, and (2) in understanding the variability in processing of the promotion of fruit and vegetables, the attention for, and reinforcing value of, these foods, as well as subsequent intake.

Conclusion

In order to improve children's eating behavior and reduce the number of children who become overweight or obese, it is necessary to test effective methods to make healthy foods more appealing and subsequently increase the intake of these food products, preferably substituting high-fat, sugar, and sodium foods. The main aim of this chapter was to show a newly designed overarching theoretical model that explains and predicts *whether, how, when*, and for *whom* food-promoting techniques increase young children's fruit and vegetable intake, in both the short and long term. Existing evidence shows that food advertising affects eating behavior among children, but most research has focused on the effects of unhealthy food advertising on children's eating behavior. The proposed Promotion of Healthy Food Model provides a framework that links up existing empirical evidence on how food promotion techniques influence eating behavior, and provides future research questions as well as intervention opportunities.

The newly developed comprehensive theoretical model can be used to create new strategies and programs that can be part of a greater food transformation, as has been proposed by a large group of scientific researchers to improve sustainable and healthy dietary behavior (Willett et al., 2019). Insights obtained from the current project can be transferred to a wide variety of healthy products, for example, those that improve the intake of water. The theoretical model has the potential to provide society, policy makers, and scholars from a great variety of scientific disciplines (e.g., health and nutrition science; consumer, neuropsychology, and developmental psychology; pediatrics; and communication science) who make it a high priority to tackle childhood obesity (WHO, 2017) with important insights in improving the intake of healthy foods among different groups of children. Multiple scholars from various disciplines are examining different methods to improve dietary intake to improve the risks of developing childhood obesity, health, and mental well-being. Insights gleaned through the proposed theoretical model could improve these methods and intervention techniques. Moreover, the theoretical model provides an increased understanding of how healthy food promotion influences dietary intake among children from different backgrounds, and which interventions are needed to improve dietary intake among children.

A great number of studies have shown that diets which are largely based on plants are high in micronutrient density, decrease the probability of heart disease and diabetes, and lead to improvements in glycemic control, weight loss, longer-term acceptability and sustainability, and reduction in multiple forms of cancer (Wright, Wilson, Smith, Duncan, & McHugh, 2017). In addition, the production of fruit and vegetables is more sustainable since it generally requires less land, energy, and water resources than diets that are high in animal products (Oppenlander, 2013; Willett et al., 2019). Therefore, a new and innovative political philosophy that influences all levels of society in order to improve healthy lifestyles is very much needed. One such political philosophy, one that has become highly relevant and has been implemented increasingly, mostly referred to as libertarian paternalism (Thaler & Sunstein, 2003), is the philosophical idea that it is possible and legitimate for private and public institutions to influence behavior in a positive way, while at the same time respecting freedom of choice (Loewenstein, Brennan, & Volpp, 2007; Vallgårda, 2018). Efforts should be directed towards leveraging decision errors, which ordinarily have a detrimental effect on people but with the right modification could also result in positive outcomes, to reverse the trend of increased (childhood) obesity. Such a strategy will require bold action by policymakers, however, in increasing the promotion of healthier foods as well as relying on evidence-based interventions to help children defend themselves against commercial messages promoting unhealthy food intake. This can be done by reorganizing the relevant choice architecture, referring to an alteration of the context in which decisions are made. For example, a nudge is the result of choice architecture which leads to a predictable change in behavior, without limiting choices or changing economic incentives (Thaler & Sunstein, 2009).

In the food marketing domain, some experts counsel against using the same promotional techniques that are used by food companies that market unhealthy foods, because of their potential to undermine intrinsic motivation to obtain and consume healthier foods. As a result, using such techniques may backfire for some children (Folkvord et al., 2013). Therefore, political and societal discussions should be held in order to create more public awareness and generate support for implementing contextual modifications.

Political and societal debate on these and related issues is imperative. The strategies applied to date by governments, schools, parents, and other stakeholders concerning the nutrition of children knowingly or unknowingly affect children's dietary behavior in ways that are positive (e.g., increased dietary variety and intake of healthier foods, decreased pickiness and neophobia), negative (e.g., decreased intake of healthier foods, increased levels of neophobia), or simply have no effect on children's eating behavior at all. Given the great focus on public health, as well as parents' controlling approach when it concerns their children's food intake, it is vital to rethink and reflect upon different and effective approaches to changing children's eating behavior.

References

Alissa, E. M., & Ferns, G. A. (2017). Dietary fruits and vegetables and cardiovascular diseases risk. *Critical Reviews in Food Science and Nutrition, 57*(9), 1950–1962.

Anschutz, D. J., Engels, R. C., & Van Strien, T. (2009). Side effects of television food commercials on concurrent nonadvertised sweet snack food intakes in young children. *The American Journal of Clinical Nutrition, 89*(5), 1328–1333.

Anschutz, D. J., Engels, R. C., & Van Strien, T. (2010). Maternal encouragement to be thin moderates the effect of commercials on children's snack food intake. *Appetite, 55*(1), 117–123.

Anzman-Frasca, S., Savage, J. S., Marini, M. E., Fisher, J. O., & Birch, L. L. (2012). Repeated exposure and associative conditioning promote preschool children's liking of vegetables. *Appetite, 58*(2), 543–553.

Aune, D., Giovannucci, E., Boffetta, P., Fadnes, L. T., Keum, N., Norat, T., . . . & Tonstad, S. (2017). Fruit and vegetable intake and the risk of cardiovascular disease, total cancer and all-cause mortality—a systematic review and dose–response meta-analysis of prospective studies. *International Journal of Epidemiology, 46*(3), 1029–1056.

Baldassarre, F., & Campo, R. (2015). A character a day keeps the fruit on display: The influence of cartoon characters on preschoolers' preference for healthy food. *International Journal of Markets and Business Systems, 1*(3), 260–274.

Bazzano, L. A., He, J., Ogden, L. G., Loria, C. M., Vupputuri, S., Myers, L., & Whelton, P. K. (2002). Fruit and vegetable intake and risk of cardiovascular disease in US adults: The first National Health and Nutrition Examination Survey epidemiologic follow-up study. *The American Journal of Clinical Nutrition, 76*(1), 93–99.

Berridge, K. C., & Kringelbach, M. L. (2015). Pleasure systems in the brain. *Neuron, 86*(3), 646–664.

Berridge, K. C., & Robinson, T. E. (2003). Parsing reward. *Trends in Neurosciences, 26*(9), 507–513.

Birch, L. L. (1999). Development of food preferences. *Annual Review of Nutrition, 19*(1), 41–62.

Boon, B., Stroebe, W., Schut, H., & Jansen, A. (1998). Food for thought: Cognitive regulation of food intake. *British Journal of Health Psychology, 3*(1), 27–40.

Boswell, R. G., & Kober, H. (2016). Food cue reactivity and craving predict eating and weight gain: A meta-analytic review. *Obesity Reviews, 17*(2), 159–177.

Boyland, E. J., & Halford, J. C. (2013). Television advertising and branding. Effects on eating behaviour and food preferences in children. *Appetite, 62*, 236–241.

Boyland, E. J., Kavanagh-Safran, M., & Halford, J. C. (2015). Exposure to 'healthy' fast food meal bundles in television advertisements promotes liking for fast food but not healthier choices in children. *British Journal of Nutrition, 113*(6), 1012–1018.

Boyland, E. J., Nolan, S., Kelly, B., Tudur-Smith, C., Jones, A., Halford, J. C., & Robinson, E. (2016). Advertising as a cue to consume: a systematic review and meta-analysis of the effects of acute exposure to unhealthy food and nonalcoholic beverage advertising on intake in children and adults, 2. *The American Journal of Clinical Nutrition, 103*(2), 519–533.

Bruce, A. S., Lepping, R. J., Bruce, J. M., Cherry, J. B. C., Martin, L. E., Davis, A. M., . . . & Savage, C. R. (2013). Brain responses to food logos in obese and healthy weight children. *The Journal of Pediatrics, 162*(4), 759–764.

Cairns, G., Angus, K., Hastings, G., & Caraher, M. (2013). Systematic reviews of the evidence on the nature, extent and effects of food marketing to children. A retrospective summary. *Appetite, 62*, 209–215.

Carnell, S., Benson, L., Driggin, E., & Kolbe, L. (2014). Parent feeding behavior and child appetite: Associations depend on feeding style. *International Journal of Eating Disorders, 47*(7), 705–709.

Carter, B. L., & Tiffany, S. T. (1999). Meta-analysis of cue-reactivity in addiction research. *Addiction, 94*(3), 327–340

Caton, S. J., Blundell, P., Ahern, S. M., Nekitsing, C., Olsen, A., Møller, P., . . . & Issanchou, S. (2014). Learning to eat vegetables in early life: the role of timing, age and individual eating traits. *PloS One, 9*(5), e97609.

Chandon, P., & Wansink, B. (2012). Does food marketing need to make us fat? A review and solutions. *Nutrition Reviews, 70*(10), 571–593.

Cooke, L. J., Chambers, L. C., Añez, E. V., Croker, H. A., Boniface, D., Yeomans, M. R., & Wardle, J. (2011). Eating for pleasure or profit: The effect of incentives on children's enjoyment of vegetables. *Psychological Science, 22*(2), 190–196.

De Cock, N., Van Lippevelde, W., Goossens, L., De Clercq, B., Vangeel, J., Lachat, C., . . . & Maes, L. (2016). Sensitivity to reward and adolescents' unhealthy snacking and drinking behavior: The role of hedonic eating styles and availability. *International Journal of Behavioral Nutrition and Physical Activity, 13*(1), 17.

DeCosta, P., Møller, P., Frøst, M. B., & Olsen, A. (2017). Changing children's eating behaviour: A review of experimental research. *Appetite, 113*, 327–357.

de Droog, S. M., Buijzen, M., & Valkenburg, P. M. (2014). Enhancing children's vegetable consumption using vegetable-promoting picture books. The impact of interactive shared reading and character–product congruence. *Appetite, 73*, 73–80.

De Droog, S. M., Valkenburg, P. M., & Buijzen, M. (2010). Using brand characters to promote young children's liking of and purchase requests for fruit. *Journal of Health Communication, 16*(1), 79–89.

Dovey, T. M., Taylor, L., Stow, R., Boyland, E. J., & Halford, J. C. (2011). Responsiveness to healthy television (TV) food advertisements/commercials is only evident in children under the age of seven with low food neophobia. *Appetite, 56*(2), 440–446.

Ferriday, D., & Brunstrom, J. M. (2011). 'I just can't help myself': Effects of food-cue exposure in overweight and lean individuals. *International Journal of Obesity*, *35*(1), 142.

Fildes, A., van Jaarsveld, C. H., Cooke, L., Wardle, J., & Llewellyn, C. H. (2016). Common genetic architecture underlying young children's food fussiness and liking for vegetables and fruit–3. *The American Journal of Clinical Nutrition*, *103*(4), 1099–1104.

Fisher, C., Nicholas, P., & Marshall, W. (2011). Cooking in schools: Rewarding teachers for inspiring adolescents to make healthy choices. *Nutrition Bulletin*, *36*(1), 120–123.

Folkvord, F., Anastasiadou, D. T., & Anschütz, D. (2017). Memorizing fruit: The effect of a fruit memory-game on children's fruit intake. *Preventive Medicine Reports*, *5*, 106–111.

Folkvord, F., Anschütz, D. J., Boyland, E., Kelly, B., & Buijzen, M. (2016). Food advertising and eating behavior in children. *Current Opinion in Behavioral Sciences*, *9*, 26–31.

Folkvord, F., Anschütz, D. J., Buijzen, M., & Valkenburg, P. M. (2013). The effect of playing advergames that promote energy-dense snacks or fruit on actual food intake among children. *The American Journal of Clinical Nutrition*, *97*(2), 239–245.

Folkvord, F., Anschütz, D. J., Nederkoorn, C., Westerik, H., & Buijzen, M. (2014). Impulsivity, "advergames," and food intake. *Pediatrics*, *133*(6), 1007–1012.

Folkvord, F., Anschütz, D. J., Wiers, R. W., & Buijzen, M. (2015). The role of attentional bias in the effect of food advertising on actual food intake among children. *Appetite*, *84*, 251–258.

Folkvord, F., & Laguna-Camacho, A. (2019). The effect of a memory-game with images of vegetables on children's vegetable intake: An experimental study. *Appetite*, *134*, 120–124.

Folkvord, F., Veling, H., & Hoeken, H. (2016). Targeting implicit approach reactions to snack food in children: Effects on intake. *Health Psychology*, *35*(8), 919.

Forwood, S. E., Ahern, A. L., Hollands, G. J., Ng, Y. L., & Marteau, T. M. (2015). Priming healthy eating. You can't prime all the people all of the time. *Appetite*, *89*, 93–102.

Galbraith-Emami, S., & Lobstein, T. (2013). The impact of initiatives to limit the advertising of food and beverage products to children: A systematic review. *Obesity Reviews*, *14*(12), 960–974.

Gearhardt, A. N., Yokum, S., Stice, E., Harris, J. L., & Brownell, K. D. (2014). Relation of obesity to neural activation in response to food commercials. *Social Cognitive and Affective Neuroscience*, *9*(7), 932–938.

Gilbert-Diamond, D., Li, Z., Adachi-Mejia, A. M., McClure, A. C., & Sargent, J. D. (2014). Association of a television in the bedroom with increased adiposity gain in a nationally representative sample of children and adolescents. *JAMA Pediatrics*, *168*(5), 427–434.

Halford, J. C., Boyland, E. J., Hughes, G. M., Stacey, L., McKean, S., & Dovey, T. M. (2008). Beyond-brand effect of television food advertisements on food choice in children: The effects of weight status. *Public Health Nutrition*, *11*(9), 897–904.

Hanks, A. S., Just, D. R., & Brumberg, A. (2016). Marketing vegetables in eleentary school cafeterias to increase uptake. *Pediatrics*, e20151720.

Harris, J. L., LoDolce, M., Dembek, C., & Schwartz, M. B. (2015). Sweet promises: Candy advertising to children and implications for industry self-regulation. *Appetite*, *95*, 585–592.

Hofmann, W., Rauch, W., & Gawronski, B. (2007). And deplete us not into temptation: Automatic attitudes, dietary restraint, and self-regulatory resources as determinants of eating behavior. *Journal of Experimental Social Psychology*, *43*(3), 497–504.

Joshipura, K. J., Hu, F. B., Manson, J. E., Stampfer, M. J., Rimm, E. B., Speizer, F. E., . . . & Willett, W. C. (2001). The effect of fruit and vegetable intake on risk for coronary heart disease. *Annals of Internal Medicine*, *134*(12), 1106–1114.

Just, D. R., & Price, J. (2013). Using incentives to encourage healthy eating in children. *Journal of Human Resources, 48*(4), 855–872.

Kaikkonen, J. E., Mikkilä, V., Magnussen, C. G., Juonala, M., Viikari, J. S., & Raitakari, O. T. (2013). Does childhood nutrition influence adult cardiovascular disease risk? Insights from the Young Finns Study. *Annals of Medicine, 45*(2), 120–128.

Kakoschke, N., Kemps, E., & Tiggemann, M. (2014). Attentional bias modification encourages healthy eating. *Eating Behaviors, 15*(1), 120–124.

Karnik, S., & Kanekar, A. (2012). Childhood obesity: a global public health crisis. *International Journal of Preventive Medicine, 3*(1), 1–7.

Lake, A., & Townshend, T. (2006). Obesogenic environments: Exploring the built and food environments. *The Journal of the Royal Society for the Promotion of Health, 126*(6), 262–267.

Langford, R., Bonell, C., Komro, K., Murphy, S., Magnus, D., Waters, E., . . . & Campbell, R. (2017). The health promoting schools framework: Known unknowns and an agenda for future research. *Health Education & Behavior, 44*(3), 463–475.

Lobstein, T., Jackson-Leach, R., Moodie, M. L., Hall, K. D., Gortmaker, S. L., Swinburn, B. A., . . . & McPherson, K. (2015). Child and adolescent obesity: Part of a bigger picture. *The Lancet, 385*(9986), 2510–2520.

Lock, K., Pomerleau, J., Causer, L., Altmann, D. R., & McKee, M. (2005). The global burden of disease attributable to low consumption of fruit and vegetables: Implications for the global strategy on diet. *Bulletin of the World Health Organization, 83*, 100–108.

Loewenstein, G., Brennan, T., & Volpp, K. G. (2007). Asymmetric paternalism to improve health behaviors. *JAMA, 298*(20), 2415–2417.

Mackenbach, J. P., Stirbu, I., Roskam, A. J. R., Schaap, M. M., Menvielle, G., Leinsalu, M., & Kunst, A. E. (2008). Socioeconomic inequalities in health in 22 European countries. *New England Journal of Medicine, 358*(23), 2468–2481.

Nederkoorn, C., Smulders, F. T. Y., & Jansen, A. (2000). Cephalic phase responses, craving and food intake in normal subjects. *Appetite, 35*(1), 45–55.

Ness, A. R., & Powles, J. W. (1997). Fruit and vegetables, and cardiovascular disease: A review. *International Journal of Epidemiology, 26*(1), 1–13.

Nijs, I. M., Franken, I. H., & Muris, P. (2010). Food-related Stroop interference in obese and normal-weight individuals: Behavioral and electrophysiological indices. *Eating Behaviors, 11*(4), 258–265.

Nijs, I. M., Muris, P., Euser, A. S., & Franken, I. H. (2010). Differences in attention to food and food intake between overweight/obese and normal-weight females under conditions of hunger and satiety. *Appetite, 54*(2), 243–254.

Norman, J., Kelly, B., McMahon, A. T., Boyland, E., Baur, L. A., Chapman, K., . . . & Bauman, A. (2018). Children's self-regulation of eating provides no defense against television and online food marketing. *Appetite, 125*, 438–444.

Oliver, J. (2018). *Jamie's plan to halve childhood obesity by 2030 in the UK.* Retrieved from: https://www.jamieoliver.com/news-and-features/features/jamies-plan-to-tackle-childhood-obesity/ Accessed on 29-12-2018.

Oppenlander, R. (2013). *Food choice and sustainability: Why buying local, eating less meat, and taking baby steps won't work.* Minneapolis, MN: Langdon Street Press.

Papies, E. K. (2016). Health goal priming as a situated intervention tool: How to benefit from nonconscious motivational routes to health behaviour. *Health Psychology Review, 10*(4), 408–424.

Pearce, A., Kirk, C., Cummins, S., Collins, M., Elliman, D., Connolly, A. M., & Law, C. (2009). Gaining children's perspectives: A multiple method approach to explore environmental influences on healthy eating and physical activity. *Health & Place, 15*(2), 614–621.

Pempek, T. A., & Calvert, S. L. (2009). Tipping the balance: use of advergames to promote consumption of nutritious foods and beverages by low-income African American children. *Archives of Pediatrics & Adolescent Medicine, 163*(7), 633–637.

Provencher, V., Polivy, J., & Herman, C. P. (2009). Perceived healthiness of food. If it's healthy, you can eat more! *Appetite, 52*(2), 340–344.

Rangel, A. (2013). Regulation of dietary choice by the decision-making circuitry. *Nature Neuroscience, 16*(12), 1717.

Rapuano, K. M., Huckins, J. F., Sargent, J. D., Heatherton, T. F., & Kelley, W. M. (2015). Individual differences in reward and somatosensory-motor brain regions correlate with adiposity in adolescents. *Cerebral Cortex, 26*(6), 2602–2611.

Rapuano, K. M., Zieselman, A. L., Kelley, W. M., Sargent, J. D., Heatherton, T. F., & Gilbert-Diamond, D. (2017). Genetic risk for obesity predicts nucleus accumbens size and responsivity to real-world food cues. *Proceedings of the National Academy of Sciences, 114*(1), 160–165.

Rooney, C., McKinley, M. C., & Woodside, J. V. (2013). The potential role of fruit and vegetables in aspects of psychological well-being: A review of the literature and future directions. *Proceedings of the Nutrition Society, 72*(4), 420–432.

Sandström, B., Marckmann, P., & Bindslev, N. (1992). An eight-month controlled study of a low-fat high-fibre diet: Effects on blood lipids and blood pressure in healthy young subjects. *European Journal of Clinical Nutrition, 46*(2), 95–109.

Sheeran, P., Gollwitzer, P. M., & Bargh, J. A. (2013). Nonconscious processes and health. *Health Psychology, 32*(5), 460.

Shepherd, J., Harden, A., Rees, R., Brunton, G., Garcia, J., Oliver, S., & Oakley, A. (2006). Young people and healthy eating: A systematic review of research on barriers and facilitators. *Health Education Research, 21*(2), 239–257.

Shrewsbury, V., & Wardle, J. (2008). Socioeconomic status and adiposity in childhood: A systematic review of cross-sectional studies 1990–2005. *Obesity, 16*(2), 275–284.

Spear, B. A., Barlow, S. E., Ervin, C., Ludwig, D. S., Saelens, B. E., Schetzina, K. E., & Taveras, E. M. (2007). Recommendations for treatment of child and adolescent overweight and obesity. *Pediatrics, 120*(Supplement 4), S254–S288.

Spence, A. C., Campbell, K. J., Lioret, S., & McNaughton, S. A. (2018). Early childhood vegetable, fruit, and discretionary food intakes do not meet dietary guidelines, but do show socioeconomic differences and tracking over time. *Journal of the Academy of Nutrition and Dietetics, 118*(9), 1634–1643.

Stevenson, C., Doherty, G., Barnett, J., Muldoon, O. T., & Trew, K. (2007). Adolescents' views of food and eating: Identifying barriers to healthy eating. *Journal of Adolescence, 30*(3), 417–434.

Swinburn, B., Egger, G., & Raza, F. (1999). Dissecting obesogenic environments: The development and application of a framework for identifying and prioritizing environmental interventions for obesity. *Preventive Medicine, 29*(6), 563–570.

Szymlek-Gay, E. A., Ferguson, E. L., Heath, A. L. M., Gray, A. R., & Gibson, R. S. (2009). Food-based strategies improve iron status in toddlers: A randomized controlled trial. *The American Journal of Clinical Nutrition, 90*(6), 1541–1551.

Thaler, R. H., & Sunstein, C. R. (2003). Libertarian paternalism. *American Economic Review, 93*(2), 175–179.

Thaler, R. H., & Sunstein, C. R. (2009). *Nudge: Improving decisions about health, wealth, and happiness*. London: Penguin.

Vallgårda, S. (2018). Childhood obesity policies – mighty concerns, meek reactions. *Obesity Reviews, 19*(3), 295–301.

Vandevijvere, S., Chow, C. C., Hall, K. D., Umali, E., & Swinburn, B. A. (2015). Increased food energy supply as a major driver of the obesity epidemic: A global analysis. *Bulletin of the World Health Organization, 93*, 446–456.

van't Riet, J., Sijtsema, S. J., Dagevos, H., & de Bruijn, G. J. (2011). The importance of habits in eating behaviour. An overview and recommendations for future research. *Appetite, 57*(3), 585–596.

Volkow, N. D., Wang, G. J., & Baler, R. D. (2011). Reward, dopamine and the control of food intake: implications for obesity. *Trends in Cognitive Sciences, 15*(1), 37–46.

Volkow, N. D., Wang, G. J., Fowler, J. S., & Telang, F. (2008). Overlapping neuronal circuits in addiction and obesity: evidence of systems pathology. *Philosophical Transactions of the Royal Society of London B: Biological Sciences, 363*(1507), 3191–3200.

Willett, W. C. (1994). Diet and health: what should we eat? *Science, 264*(5158), 532–537.

Willett, W., Rockström, J., Loken, B., Springmann, M., Lang, T., Vermeulen, S., . . . & Jonell, M. (2019). Food in the Anthropocene: The EAT–Lancet Commission on healthy diets from sustainable food systems. *The Lancet, 393*(10170), 447–492.

World Health Organization (WHO) (2017). *Global strategy on diet, physical activity and health.* Retrieved from: https://www.who.int/dietphysicalactivity/childhood/en/ on February 25th, 2019.

Wright, N., Wilson, L., Smith, M., Duncan, B., & McHugh, P. (2017). The BROAD study: A randomised controlled trial using a whole food plant-based diet in the community for obesity, ischaemic heart disease or diabetes. *Nutrition & Diabetes, 7*(3), e256.

Zahm, D. S. (2000). An integrative neuroanatomical perspective on some subcortical substrates of adaptive responding with emphasis on the nucleus accumbens. *Neuroscience & Biobehavioral Reviews, 24*(1), 85–105.

INDEX

Note: References in *italics* are to figures.

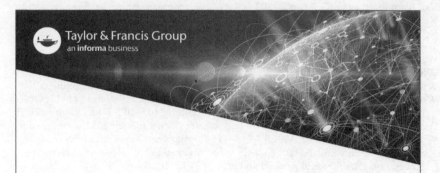